# The Power of Ayurveda

# THE POWER OF AYURVEDA

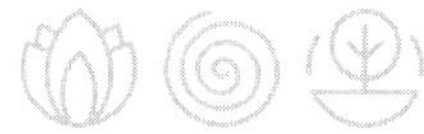

## Science-Backed Wisdom for Wellness, Vitality, and Longevity

Ulli Allmendinger

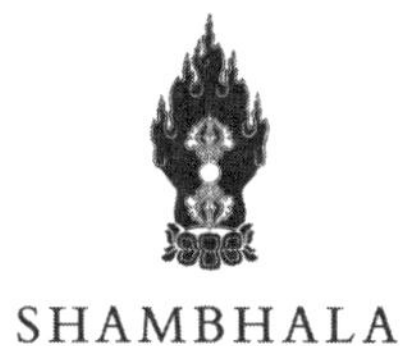

SHAMBHALA

Shambhala Publications, Inc.
2129 13th Street
Boulder, Colorado 80302
www.shambhala.com



Cover art: shopplaywood / stock.adobe.com
Cover design: Lauren Michelle Smith
Interior design: Gopa & Ted2, Inc.



9 8 7 6 5 4 3 2 1

First Edition
Printed in the United States of America

Shambhala Publications makes every effort to print on acid-free, recycled paper.
Shambhala Publications is distributed worldwide by Penguin Random House, Inc., and its subsidiaries.

Library of Congress Cataloging-in-Publication Data
Names: Allmendinger, Ulli author
Title: The power of ayurveda: science-backed wisdom for wellness, vitality, and longevity / Ulli Allmendinger.
Description: First edition. | Boulder, Colorado: Shambhala Publications, Inc, [2026] | Includes bibliographical references and index. |
Identifiers: LCCN 2025020504 | ISBN 9781645474333 trade paperback
Subjects: LCSH: Medicine, Ayurvedic
Classification: LCC R605 .A587 2026
LC record available at https://lccn.loc.gov/2025020504

The authorized representative in the EU for product safety and compliance is eucomply OÜ, Pärnu mnt 139b-14, 11317 Tallinn, Estonia, hello@eucompliancepartner.com.

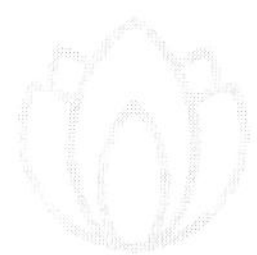

# Contents

# Introduction: Ancient Is the New Cutting Edge

If Ayurveda were a religion Nature would be its Goddess,
and overindulgence would be the sole sin She would punish.
Ayurveda is meant to allow you to enjoy the pleasures of life up
to the point that such enjoyment interferes with your health.
Full-time gratification is in fact bondage, because the more we
consume the more we become captives of our consumption.
—Dr. Robert Svoboda

## My Journey

Flashback. It is the year 2002, and I am in New York City. I have been in the city for two years, first studying at New York University, then working as a journalist and public relations specialist. New York had always fascinated me. It was larger than life, a city with a huge ego but charming and seductive nevertheless—big, beautiful, crazy, vibrant, and challenging. I fell in love with New York the moment I arrived. We just clicked. I blended in seamlessly, always on the go, running from deadline to deadline, catching the latest art shows, socializing, and mingling. I would not miss a party, yet I'd still get up at six the next morning for my run or a round of Ashtanga yoga. But I also noticed that I was getting increasingly fatigued. I got sick frequently, had trouble sleeping at night, and was constantly feeling cold. Largely I ignored it. My mind was telling me that I was a picture of health. After all, I was exercising, I didn't smoke or drink coffee, and I ate a vegan, almost raw diet mostly based on fruits and vegetables. Yet I lost weight, got skinnier, and had night sweats and infrequent anxiety attacks. When friends suggested that I see an acupuncturist, I reluctantly agreed.

### *I Was Addicted to My Imbalances*

It was my first introduction to holistic, mind-body medicine. I remember, at my first appointment, the Chinese doctor asked me what I had for breakfast every day, and I proudly told him that it was either nothing, a big fruit salad, or a smoothie on the go. He just shook his head and then talked to me about the energetics of food and qualities such as warming or cooling, building or cleansing. He suggested I try warm oatmeal with cinnamon instead and see how I feel. My mind was fighting, but I was intrigued. Since I was already hooked on yoga and had heard about Ayurveda as yoga's sister science, I bought *A Life of Balance* by Maya Tiwari, an international teacher of Ayurveda and the founder of the Wise Earth School of Ayurveda. The book changed my life. I realized that most of my cherished habits such as running, Ashtanga yoga, eating raw, and going nonstop were part of an addictive pattern that sent me more and more out of balance. I was addicted exactly to the things that would further imbalance me (and my Vata), even though superficially they were all "healthy" habits. My mind was telling me that I was feeling great, although my body was giving me the real message.

### *Slowly Deconditioning*

The deconditioning did not happen overnight, but I slowly began to connect to my body and sensations, and feel into whether a food, an activity, or a relationship was balancing and grounding or aggravating. Was it moving me to a state of calm, quiet, and peace or making me frantic, nervous, and edgy? I learned about the *doshas*—the three bioenergies that form our constitution (Vata, Pitta, and Kapha)—and started looking at foods and activities in terms of *gunas*, or qualities. Slowly I moved from raw foods to more cooked, warming, and building foods. I added healthy oils, such as ghee and coconut oil, and eventually even started to consume animal products again after having been vegan or vegetarian for almost sixteen years. Over time, most of my physical and psychological symptoms vanished. I felt stronger, more grounded, and happier than I had in years. Part of me, however, was still attracted to my life in New York—the pace, the glamour, the excitement. It took the company I worked for (at the time, I was doing public relations for a boutique arts consulting company in Chelsea) to go bankrupt, my boyfriend moving to Seattle, and a serious bike accident that left me immobile for a while to finally kick me out of New York the hard way.

### *Finding Ayurveda as a Way of Life*

Only six months after I had encountered Ayurveda, I found myself in Seattle—only to realize that a job I had lined up at a major Seattle arts museum fell through. I took it as a sign to take some time off to recuperate and figure out what I really wanted from life. By chance, I stumbled upon an Ayurvedic school in Seattle, decided to enroll, got hooked . . . and the rest is history. I still kept writing, but my focus now shifted from arts and culture to health and holistic living. I studied other types of yoga, meditated, traveled to India, met amazing teachers, and decided to do a second master's in Ayurvedic sciences. After that, I finally moved to New Mexico to study with one of the oldest and most famous Ayurveda teachers in the West, Dr. Vasant Lad. In his *gurukula* style of teaching, where students sit with the teacher and he transmits, Dr. Lad taught us much more than just medicine. He taught us about awareness, interconnectedness, and, most importantly, love. Rarely have I seen a human being so full of compassion and love for his students, his patients, and the world. He was and is a great inspiration to me, and this book is dedicated to him and all he has done to make Ayurveda flourish in the West, always not by separating it from Western medicine but respecting, using, and integrating both.

## Your Journey

With this book I want to give you a guide that is deeply steeped in the timeless wisdom that Ayurveda offers but, at the same time, radically adapted and updated to be contemporary, local, and practical. I have had the fortune of studying with amazing teachers—in the US and India—steeped in the Eastern tradition, with incredible knowledge and skill rooted firmly in the ancient texts and practices, and infused with humbleness and virtue. They gracefully and tirelessly serve their patients and students. This book is wholeheartedly based on those ancient teachings, their universal timeless truth, and the lineage of teachers. I do not want to present you with a watered-down version of this deeply rich, highly intuitive, and eloquently complex science that has a track record of more than five thousand years. Nor do I want to jump on the bandwagon of trying to use Ayurveda to fit current trends or oversimplify it. Instead, I set out to do the impossible. I want to show you that ancient is actually cutting-edge.

## Ancient Is the New Cutting Edge

Let me explain. By now you may all be familiar with ginger and turmeric as amazing anti-inflammatory spices. Your dentist may even have told you to scrape your tongue or do oil pulling because these practices are now considered as essential for oral health as brushing your teeth. And if you have ever done a detox, you probably included water or coffee enemas and dry-brushing to cleanse the liver and colon and boost lymphatic flow. But did you know that all these common practices are ancient, time-tested Ayurvedic routines? How about the new science of circadian medicine, which revealed that each organ in our body has its own internal clock that helps regulate its function and works in conjunction with the body's overall circadian rhythm? For millennia, Chinese medicine and Ayurveda have based treatments on the idea of cyclical energy flow throughout the day and night, where peak energy times are correlated with organs. They have used those times for therapies, administering herbs, and to guide lifestyle practices that support the health of each organ as well as the organism.

### *Time-Tested Wisdom Instead of Sound Bites*

Profound, ancient, and time-tested wisdom is so desperately needed nowadays where diet, supplements, and exercise fads are changing weekly, and we are continuously bombarded by sound bites of half-cooked knowledge. There is one caveat, however. If the ancient wisdom of Ayurveda wants to remain cutting-edge, its application (not the underlying truth!) also needs to evolve and adapt from five thousand years ago to the here and now. After all, by definition, Ayurveda is a living science (*ayu*, "life"; *veda*, "science"). I want you to be able to use Ayurveda to make sense of your life today. And I want you to be inspired to use it as a living body of knowledge that you can directly apply to take your health, nutrition, exercise routine, work, and relationships to a new level.

## How This Book Works

I wanted this book to be practical. After all, Ayurveda is not just a system of medicine, a bunch of herbs or supplements, or a body treatment you get at the spa. It is, by definition, a science of life and, as such, a practical, hands-on way of living. Ayurveda is a lifestyle. Therefore I decided to divide this book into three sections. In the first part, I give you the basics. It may at first seem a little boring or overwhelming, but bear with me. Part one is a little bit like learning a new language. You get to know the Ayurvedic terminology and its basic theory—in short, the framework. You learn how to better understand the world and yourself through the lens of Ayurveda. Most importantly, you get to know your unique skills and assets, as well as your weak spots. Knowledge is power.

### *Learn the Three Crucial Factors for Living Long*

From the perspective of Ayurvedic physiology, there are three essential factors for living your best and living long that we will explore together in this book. And you already have them built in from birth because each of them is related to the essential power of one of the Ayurvedic doshas: Flow (Vata), Transformation (Pitta), and Regeneration (Kapha). In other words, what makes or breaks your health and vitality is how well you are attuned to the circadian rhythm or the daily and seasonal doshic waves (Flow); how strong your digestive and metabolic power is (Transformation); and how resilient you are to physical and mental stressors (Regeneration).

### *Your Step-By-Step Guided Journey Back to Health*

In the first part of the book, I dive deep into the workings of these three ancient secrets to health. I want you to really understand those factors so that you are primed and equipped optimally before you embark on the Ayurveda 2.0 journey. This is the second part of the book, in which I offer very practical, hands-on information to guide you step by step to health, vitality, and wellness. You will see that far from being an excruciatingly exhausting marathon or an uphill battle, it is a rather pleasant and intuitive stroll through the beautiful and rich landscape of an Ayurvedic way of life. First, we fine-tune the way you *flow* by resetting your circadian and doshic rhythm. Then we optimize the way you *transform* through igniting digestion and metabolic activity. And lastly, we get you to *regenerate* by detoxing lymph (*rasa*) and supporting the nervous system so you can enjoy greater physical and mental resilience.

The fourth part of the book is devoted to supporting your journey in the kitchen. I will show you that with a few simple tricks, you can transform your cooking into medicine. Ayurvedic cooking does not have to be expensive or complicated. Neither does it have to always be Indian food. It simply means high-quality, local, and seasonal ingredients that are prepared in a way that is most nourishing, digestible, and delicious—for your unique metabolic, digestive, and doshic strength. You will find all recipes necessary for your Ayurveda journey, as well as a few bonuses that you can have on hand to easily make any meal more nutritious and digestible. In this section I invite you to enter your kitchen as an explorer and find new ways of relating to food and cooking creatively, confidently, and joyfully.

I hope you will use this book to become your own doctor or inner alchemist, optimizing your physical, mental, and spiritual health and well-being so that you can contribute to the world your unique gifts and talents.

# Part One

## Understanding Ayurveda 2.0

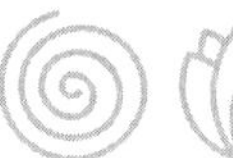  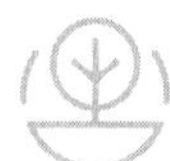

# What Is Ayurveda Today?

## Time-Tested Wisdom: The Spiritual Roots and Origins of Ayurveda

Ayurveda is often called the "mother" of all healing modalities. It is one of the oldest systems of natural healing, reaching back more than five thousand years and predating even Chinese medicine. Originating in the Vedic culture of India, Ayurveda was—at least so the texts state—actually channeled by the wise old yogis (rishis) of India as a body of timeless knowledge that would help humankind regain health, balance, and longevity at a time when disease and malaise was rampant. (If things were already pretty bad back then, I don't want to know where we stand today.) The roots of Ayurveda go back to the Vedas, the oldest sacred literature in the world that in its current form probably dates back to 1500 B.C.E., preserved by Indian priests as revelations directly from Source or Brahma (or Creator) itself. From the youngest of the Vedas, the *Atharvaveda*, Ayurveda developed and was systematized somewhere around 1000 B.C.E. I find it fascinating that while firmly rooted in Vedic belief and the culture of its time, Ayurveda developed as an empirical medical science through a process of critical thinking and clinical observation. This is largely because in the East, science is not separated from philosophy or religion; each is seen as a different but equally valid and important way of experiencing and understanding truth.

### *We Are Deeply Interconnected*

One such fundamental truth of Eastern thought and philosophy is the principle of deep interconnectivity and interdependence between us and the world around us. While Western philosophical thought is often characterized by a focus on individualism, rationalism, and objectivity, Eastern philosophy emphasizes the interconnectivity of all of life and the importance of acknowledging the whole rather than the individual parts. This concept mirrors the idea of an interwoven web of life, where each strand is connected to the others. Here, our environment (macrocosm) is just an outward expression of our body and mind (microcosm), and vice versa. Both the environment and mind-body are made up of the five elements (earth, water, fire, air, and space) and three forces: movement or flow, transformation, and regeneration. In Ayurveda, and associated with the body, these are often referred to as the doshas or bioenergies: Vata (movement or flow), Pitta (transformation), and Kapha (regeneration). All three doshas must be graciously working together for a person to experience optimal health and well-being.

### *An Oral Tradition Is Systemized*

While Ayurvedic medicine initially was passed from generation to generation in an oral tradition, organized in small verses (sutras), over time it was systematically written down. Today we have several original texts comprising its vast knowledge.[1] First, the *Charaka Samhita*, compiled approximately 1000 B.C.E., is the oldest Sanskrit text on Ayurveda; today it is often used as the main referential text for Ayurvedic doctors, especially in northern India. Second, the *Sushruta Samhita*, the first text describing surgery long before it was ever performed in the West. Third, *Ashtanga Hridayam*, compiled by the famous South Indian Ayurvedic physician Vagbhata, is a concise and succinct summary of the *Charaka Samhita*; today it is the main referential textbook for most practitioners in southern India. Throughout this book I will use quotes from these ancient texts to show you how modern and cutting-edge this ancient wisdom is.

## If I Am Not Sick, Am I Healthy? Redefining Health and Disease Through the Lens of Ayurveda

The Sanskrit word *ayur-veda* comprises two syllables: *ayu*, "life"; and *veda* or *vidya*, "science." As such, Ayurveda is not "just" a medical system for treating disease but a "science of life," the art of understanding and living life to its fullest and highest potential. To know Ayurveda means to live it. In India I recently also heard another definition, which I really love: "Ayurveda means learning to live and living to learn." With the help of Ayurveda, we are learning to better understand ourselves, the world around us, and our place in it. Only then can we live a balanced, healthy, and meaningful life. Ayurveda brings us back home to the innate wisdom that is wired into the core of each and every one of us as well as into every cell of our organism.

### *Live with Reality, Otherwise Reality Comes to Live with You*

Ayurveda is based on living in sync. According to Ayurveda, we need to cooperate with nature to ensure our well-being. I always remember the first talk I attended by Dr. Robert Svoboda, the renowned Ayurvedic physician and author who is still a great inspiration for me. It was in Seattle in 2004, and I had just embarked on my journey of learning Ayurveda. He quoted his mentor, the Aghori Vimalananda, as saying, "You have to live with reality, otherwise reality comes to live with you." If there is one saying that embodies the wisdom of Ayurveda, this is it. I probably quote this to my students and clients more than any other phrase because it clearly states that the only way to avoid suffering or disease is to align ourselves with the macro, with natural laws and the cosmos. Otherwise we suffer the consequences. For example, I can continuously stay up partying until the morning hours and sleep until noon, completely ignoring the fact that I am a diurnal being and my circadian rhythm is deeply wired into my DNA. I will in some way have to pay the debt of going against the circadian rhythm with a weakened immune system, an increased risk of heart disease and stroke, hormonal dysregulation, and a good chance of developing diabetes and obesity. Again and again we need to remind ourselves that we are intrinsically connected and interdependent with the universe, the macrocosm. What happens on the planet also happens inside our bodies. From this point of view, health is more than the dynamic balance between body, mind, and spirit; it is also about resonance with the outer environment (nature). As such, rather than just the absence of disease, health is a comprehensive and dynamic state of well-being—a well-being of all, including the earth itself.

### *Health Is More Than Not Being Sick*

He whose doshas are in balance, whose appetite (digestion) is good,
whose tissues are functioning normally, whose wastes are in balance,
and whose consciousness, mind, and senses remain full of bliss,
and he who is established in the Self, is called a healthy person.
—SUSHRUTA SAMHITA 15.38

The *Sushruta Samhita* offers a pretty comprehensive definition of health, doesn't it? Even if you are physically healthy, if your mind is imbalanced and you are full of greed, anger, or worry, you are in fact not healthy. *Sushruta Samhita* goes even one step further. If your body is strong and your mind is calm, but you are not *svastha*—"established or situated within yourself"—you are not healthy. Being situated within yourself basically means to know yourself, your essential nature, your inner strengths and weaknesses. Lately I have been thinking that *svastha* also means knowing your place on earth. We are only one small part of nature (albeit a very powerful and destructive one). We can only be truly healthy when we take our humble and rightful place again as part of, rather than ruling over, nature. Only then can we be svastha and start living in harmony with the earth and its animals, trees, oceans, and rivers.

### *All Disease Starts in the Mind*

Disease, then, according to Ayurveda, is anything less than perfect health. This can be an abnormal function of the doshas, the tissues (*dhatus*), elimination (*malas*), disturbance of mind (*manas*), or, at the utmost root, forgetting our true nature or our place on earth. From this perspective, while environmental factors, stress, lifestyle choices, or poor nutrition are all major contributing factors to disease, ultimately all disease originates from this deep misunderstanding of our essential nature. It starts in the mind. The classical texts refer to it as *prajnaparadha* (*prajna*, "intellect"; *aparadha*, "offense" or "fault"), often translated as "mistaken intellect" or "crimes against wisdom." While deep inside we know better, still we pursue things that we know are ultimately harming us and the planet, such as staying up late, eating fast foods or factory-raised animals, drinking too much coffee, smoking, or abusing alcohol. Ultimately the pursuit of pleasure rules over what the body—and the earth—can tolerate without being harmed. The more imbalanced our bodies become, the more toxins coat the cells and make proper signaling and communication impossible. Consequently the mind also becomes foggy, clouded, and less able to discern, see, and understand clearly. This is an endless vicious cycle that can only be broken when we develop a radically new understanding of ourselves.

### *A New Paradigm of Medicine*

Ultimately the Eastern concept of health and disease offers a new paradigm for medicine. In Ayurveda, just like in Chinese medicine, there is no separation between body and mind, inside and outside, nature and humans, or even individual organs and organ systems. All are beautifully and inextricably linked and connected. Thus health and healing can only happen when all these parts are healthy, communicating with each other, and functioning together. New developments in Western medicine, such as functional or systems medicine, are speaking to this point and now acknowledging what the mother of all systems medicine—Ayurveda—postulated five thousand years ago.

## Beyond Curry and Oil Massage: Nine Myths About Ayurveda

Before we embark on our journey, there are nine common myths regarding Ayurveda that I would like to address. I wanted to specifically clarify these points from the start because I got stuck there in my early years with Ayurveda, and I have encountered these misconceptions repeatedly in my twenty years of practice with clients, with students, and increasingly in (social) media.

1. **Ayurveda is Indian medicine.** Yes, Ayurveda is a medical system that originated from the Indian subcontinent and has been around

for thousands of years. But just like homeopathy is not "German medicine," even though it was founded by the German doctor Samuel Hahnemann in the nineteenth century, Ayurveda has firm roots in India and the Vedic culture of its time but it is not Indian medicine. According to the classical texts, Ayurveda is based on timeless universal truths and principles that are independent of culture and locality. Ayurveda, just like Chinese medicine, is a perennial wisdom because it is a universal healing system. It can be applied to people of all cultures and backgrounds. Ayurveda is based on the premise that health and wellness depend on a balance between the mind, body, and spirit, as well as the environment. As a natural and universal system of healing, it teaches how to bring about health and healing using different measures such as personalized diet, herbs, detoxification, and body therapies.

2. **Ayurveda is a religion.** Ayurveda is neither a mythology nor a religion but rather a highly elaborate scientific system that uses the framework of elements, gunas, and doshas to understand the human body. While it is embedded in the culture and philosophy of the Vedas and is a sister science to other Vedic disciplines such as yoga, Jyotish (Vedic astrology), and Vastu Shastra (Vedic sacred geometry), Ayurveda does not involve any faith or belief system, nor does it prescribe any specific religious practices.
3. **Ayurveda is complicated and time-consuming.** An Ayurvedic lifestyle does not have to be time-consuming. While there are some elaborate morning routines, such as self-oil massage, many Ayurvedic practices are simple and require little effort, such as drinking warm water with lemon in the morning or making lunch your biggest meal. Other practices, such as tongue scraping, can be done in just a few minutes each day. Additionally, there are many ways to incorporate Ayurvedic remedies and hacks into a busy lifestyle that can upgrade your life quality significantly.
4. **Ayurveda is expensive.** It is true that many high-end spas and luxury hotels offer expensive Ayurvedic body therapies and contribute to the myth of Ayurveda being expensive and exclusive. But Ayurveda is a simple and holistic approach to health that

is both affordable and accessible. In fact, many Ayurvedic treatments are based on nutritional and lifestyle changes or herbal remedies that can be easily implemented without the need for expensive medical treatments. In some chronic diseases with deep-seated toxicity, more complex and expensive *panchakarma* (detoxification) therapies may be recommended that are usually done in an inpatient setting. But we have many different budget options available, ranging from a few hundred dollars in small and modest Ayurvedic hospitals to several thousand in more comfortable and luxurious resorts.

5. **Ayurveda is Indian food.** Many popular cookbooks on Ayurveda heavily emphasize Indian dishes with ingredients that are often foreign to our European palate and digestion. To be clear, you don't have to consume curry, basmati rice, and lassi to benefit from Ayurvedic wisdom. Rather than a particular cuisine, Ayurvedic nutrition is more of a framework on what, when, and how to eat. This can be applied to any culture and cuisine. For the last fifteen years, I have been living and practicing in Turkey, where many ingredients such as coconut oil, split mung beans, curry leaves, and basmati rice are not readily available. But Turkey has an amazing variety of local fruits, vegetables, grains, and legumes that people there have been consuming for centuries. We can apply the principles of Ayurvedic nutrition to any cuisine and food tradition. We can also use the Ayurvedic nutritional model to include, consider, and modify or personalize a particular dietary choice such as a vegetarian, vegan, paleo, or even ketogenic diet.
6. **You must be a vegetarian to follow an Ayurvedic lifestyle.** There is a popular myth that Ayurveda means being vegetarian. It is true that Ayurveda does not recommend animal proteins for everybody. However, if you check the ancient Ayurvedic classical texts, detailed descriptions, explanations, and prescriptions for all sorts of meats are given for therapeutic purposes. While eating meat may be a personal decision based on your ethics, culture, taste preference, or habits, Ayurveda's recommendation for meat consumption is exclusively dependent on your individual

constitution, nutritional needs, and state of health. In the *Charaka Samhita*, for example, it clearly states that good-quality meats are generally strength-building (*brimhana*) but need a powerful digestive fire to digest and metabolize the heavy animal protein. Meat-based broths, on the other hand, are easy to digest and one of the most nourishing foods for a weakened or depleted body. While many people in the West tend to overconsume animal products, or consume poor-quality dairy and meat, a small amount of animal protein may be very beneficial for certain body types or in states of weakness and depletion.

7. **Ayurveda hates raw food.** While it is true that Ayurveda mainly recommends warm and cooked foods to support better digestion and absorption, raw foods also have their place. In the summer season, and in constitutions with excessive internal heat and a strong digestive fire, incorporating some amount of raw food can be beneficial. Raw foods and leafy greens are not only full of antioxidants and prana (vital energy) but also help to clear excess heat, and provide the body with vitamins, minerals, and enzymes that can help to promote balance and healing.
8. **Ayurveda condemns coffee.** Though Ayurveda would never recommend that you have several large mugs of coffee daily, under the right conditions and at the right time, you can certainly drink coffee wisely and in moderation. Ayurveda says that all plants serve a purpose, and coffee is best viewed as a (strong) medicine. An organic coffee bean is a powerhouse of polyphenol activity and antioxidants. Coffee is known to have a warming and stimulating effect; it is energizing, boosts digestion and metabolism, and raises blood pressure. These characteristics may particularly benefit Kapha body types that tend to feel heavy, sluggish, and foggy. On the contrary, if you are stressed, anxious, and overwhelmed (Vata imbalanced), coffee may not serve you well at all.
9. **Ayurveda is all about your constitution, or dosha.** Your constitution or mind-body type is, of course, always in the background and vital for getting to know yourself and developing a lifestyle based on prevention. But it plays a very small role in the treat-

ment and correction of imbalance or disease. Furthermore, it becomes a prison when we lock ourselves into a category rigidly. Twenty years ago, when I first learned I was predominantly a Vata (air) constitution, I thought I had to quit running and eat warm porridge, cooked fruit, and soup day in and out and all year round. But life is not fixed and rigid, and neither are we. Nature, elements, and doshas are continuously changing—in hourly, daily, seasonal, and lifetime cycles. So, no matter your constitutional type, your diet and lifestyle continuously evolve with the seasons and are always adjusted and synced to the here and now.

## Ayurveda 2.0: The Future Is Ancient

Before the British occupation, Ayurvedic schools and hospitals flourished in India. However, during British rule, many Ayurvedic schools and hospitals were considered "backward" and were shut down, replaced by what was then considered modern Western medicine. Recent years, however, have seen a spread of yoga—and with it, Ayurveda—throughout the Western world, which in turn led to a resurgence of Ayurveda in India. Today, many hospitals in India embrace both Western and Ayurvedic treatments.

### *Time-Tested Wisdom Instead of Half-Cooked Knowledge*

I cannot think of a better time for the revival of Ayurveda and its sister sciences yoga, Jyotish, and Vastu Shastra. We live in a time of intense fragmentation. Traditional systems of living—family, community, village, tribe—have been eroded, and many of us feel uprooted, isolated, and disconnected, despite increased technological connectivity. We have become insecure, stressed out, and overwhelmed, bombarded with sound bites of knowledge and tailored reality through television, print news, and social media. We have become knowledge junkies, but we're starving for wisdom. Ayurveda has much to offer in this respect because it is not only a vast body of knowledge about the origin and treatment of disease but also a perennial wisdom, a timeless reminder of whole-ism and balance, as well as the interconnectedness between humans, nature, and the cosmos. I like to think of Ayurveda almost like a mycelial being with an ability to tune in to and follow the invisible strands of the universe that hold us all together.

### *Ayurveda Is Alive in India*

Whenever I take my students for advanced trainings to a very special Ayurvedic healing village in Tamil Nadu, India, they are amazed to see how beautifully alive Ayurveda is there, lived authentically and consciously and practiced with effortless rigor. Deeply interwoven with spiritual practices such as daily *homa* (fire) rituals, prayers, and Hindu ceremonies, Ayurveda in India is inseparable from the rich cultural, social, and religious web it is part of. Ayurveda is alive in the villages, where grandmothers make ghee from village butter over open fire; mothers prepare fresh vegetarian meals three times a day; and *chai-wallahs* brew tea, ginger root, cardamom, and many other spices into a sweet, milky, nourishing, and delicious drink. It is also alive through the *vaidyas* (Ayurvedic doctors) who are tirelessly treating patients and teaching students, their knowledge and practices firmly rooted in the ancient classical texts. Often from childhood onward, they are familiarized with thousands of herbs and foods available that are all listed in the classics. Their treatments work in part because they are practiced on the land and in the culture they originated from.

### *Age-Old Secrets Illuminated by Cutting-Edge Science*

Yet I also have encountered many patients and students returning from a detox (*panchakarma*) in India who are overwhelmed and frustrated, with food lists that feature grains and vegetables foreign to their geography and culture, and lifestyle recommendations that are simply not practical in their modern, busy life. They struggle on for a while but then simply give up. In this light, I propose that we fully acknowledge and honor Ayurveda as the "science of life" that it is, with timeless truth and wisdom that goes beyond a particular culture and geography. We must take that truth and wisdom from the source and manage to make its practical application radically contemporary, local, and sustainable. Only then can we benefit immensely from Ayurveda's wisdom and age-old secrets, which today can also be supported and illuminated by cutting-edge modern science.

### *Traditional Wisdom Radically Updated to Be Relevant Today*

I am aware that while you are curious, you may not be interested in learning every minute and complex detail of Ayurveda as a healing system. Instead, you picked up this book because you simply want to know what you need to feel better. This is why, in this book, you will find deep Vedic thought and philosophy from the ancient texts that cut right through to fundamental truths about life and living, and you will find their wisdom applied to your life today. You will even find an Ayurvedic perspective on many contemporary trends and practices, such as intermittent fasting, the Wim Hof method, and biohacking. I address them because many of my clients are using them, and because I think that Ayurveda can offer a unique perspective and shed light on the benefits and potential dangers of these trends.

### *We Can Use Ayurveda to Navigate the Jungle We Call Modern Life*

Just like many of you, I too live a busy life. I live in a big city—Istanbul—and lead a busy practice while teaching and traveling internationally. Often I feel like my day needs at least forty hours to get through it all. And while I love my 2.5-hour Ayurvedic morning routine, I do not have time to do this every single morning. Neither do I always have the time to cook a fresh meal three times per day. Nevertheless, I can use the wisdom of Ayurveda to navigate gracefully, joyfully, and healthily through the jungle we call modern life. I invite you to do the same. The beauty of Ayurveda is that you can start right where you are and take it as far as you want. You will find that Ayurveda is not a set of rigid rules but a highly intuitive way of living that continuously evolves and deepens. With a few basic tricks, it is extremely easy to follow.

# 2

# The Matrix of the Universe

## Discover Nature Through the Lens of Ayurveda

### Fab 5: The 5 Elements as Building Blocks of Nature

According to Ayurveda, there is a fundamental relationship between nature and human beings. Just as nature is made up of the five great elements (ether, air, fire, water, earth), so is the human body. The elements are not abstract concepts but rather essential references to explain all aspects of the macrocosm (environment) and microcosm (your physical and mental condition). To understand your body, you must first understand the elements. I very much like Dr. Robert Svoboda's explanation of the elements as states of matter, where earth represents the solid state; water, the liquid state; air, the gaseous state; fire, the power to change states of any substance; and ether, as the space that contains all the others.[1]

Space is the foundation of all there is. It represents the infinite potential of creation. Air is the source of movement and communication and governs prana or chi (life force). Fire is the element of transformation and is responsible for digestion and metabolism. Water is the element of fluidity and governs lubrication, hydration, and cleansing. Earth is the element of stability and is responsible for providing the building blocks for all physical form. By understanding and balancing the five elements, we learn to tap into their power and wisdom.

#### Ether/Space (*Akasha*)

Essence: Container (of all other elements)
Qualities: Expansive, clear, light, subtle, and soft
Energy: Nuclear energy

| | |
|---|---|
| Sense: | Sound and hearing (because sound travels in space) |
| Physical: | Spaces in the body such as mouth, sinuses, gastrointestinal (GI) tract |
| Mental: | Freedom, consciousness |
| Imbalance: | Loneliness, separation, isolation |

### Air (*Vayu*)

| | |
|---|---|
| Essence: | Movement |
| Qualities: | Cold, light, subtle, clear, mobile, rough, and dry |
| Energy: | Electrical energy (friction) |
| Sense: | Touch (because you feel the wind through the touch of the skin) |
| Physical: | Gaseous exchange in the lungs; the beating of the heart; and the movement of the limbs |
| Mental: | Movement of thought and intentionality; happiness, joy, and enthusiasm |
| Imbalance: | Fear, anxiety, hyperactivity |

### Fire (*Tejas*)

| | |
|---|---|
| Essence: | Heat and transformation |
| Qualities: | Hot, dry, light, subtle, and sharp |
| Energy: | Radiant energy |
| Sense: | Eyes and seeing (because you perceive all forms and light through the eyes) |
| Physical: | Digestive enzymes, body temperature, and neurotransmitters |
| Mental: | Attention, understanding, intelligence |
| Imbalance: | Anger, envy, criticism |

### Water (*Apas*)

| | |
|---|---|
| Essence: | Binding and cohesion |
| Qualities: | Cool, liquid, dull, soft, and heavy |
| Energy: | Chemical energy |
| Sense: | Tongue and taste (because without saliva, we would not experience taste and flavor) |

| | |
|---|---|
| Physical: | Water in the body is found almost everywhere: in the cells as cytoplasm, as the liquid aspect of blood, sweat, and urine |
| Mental: | Contentment, love, compassion |
| Imbalance: | Attachment, stickiness, clinging |

**EARTH (*PRITHVI*)**

| | |
|---|---|
| Essence: | Grounding and stability |
| Qualities: | Heavy, dull, static, dense, gross, and hard |
| Energy: | Mechanical energy |
| Sense: | Nose and smell (because through smell we perceive the subtle qualities of physical substances) |
| Physical: | Body mass: bones, muscles, fat tissue |
| Mental: | Support, grounding |
| Imbalance: | Rigidity, depression |

You can see that the five elements are present on all levels of our physiology and psychology. They are even the fundamental building blocks of each individual cell. Within each cell, the cell membrane is earth; the cytoplasm is water; nucleic acid and other chemical components are fire; the movement and activity of the cell is air; and the cellular vacuoles are space.

## Team Twenty: Gunas, or the Character of Things

According to Ayurveda, everything in the universe, including the human body, is made up of the five elements. These elements have certain qualities, or gunas (from the Sanskrit root *gun*, "to count, multiply"). Air, for example, is light, cool, and dry, whereas water is soft, liquid, and dull. Gunas allow us to describe the inherent potential of any substance in the universe. It is not just theory but very practical in its application, not only for treatment purposes but also for understanding the effect of certain foods or lifestyle habits on the body.

Ayurveda lists ten pairs of opposites, or twenty qualities, that function together. These are binary opposites. In Chinese medical terms, it is the theory of yin and yang. The whole universe, including our own bodies, can be seen as a never-ending pulsation of expansion and contraction, descension and ascension, yin and yang, the two polar complementing energies.

| | |
|---|---|
| Cold | Hot |
| Oily, moist | Dry |
| Heavy | Light |
| Slow, dull | Sharp |
| Slimy, smooth | Rough |
| Dense | Liquid |
| Soft | Hard |
| Gross | Subtle |
| Static | Mobile |
| Sticky, cloudy | Clear |

Anything in the universe—not only substances but also thoughts or actions—can be described in terms of qualities. For example, a chair is cool, dry, heavy, hard, and static. Coffee is hot, drying, light, sharp, subtle, mobile, and clear. Yogurt is cold, oily, heavy, dull, smooth, dense, soft, and cloudy. Running is hot, light, rough, and mobile.

### *Gunas Are the Most Underrated Concept of Ayurveda Today*

We will come back to the gunas over and over again. They are, in my opinion, one of the most underrepresented aspects of Ayurveda today, yet they are vitally important if we want to understand the effect of food, exercise, lifestyle, herbal medicine, and thoughts on our bodies and minds. In Ayurveda, the gunas serve as a diagnostic tool, clinical barometer, and therapeutic guide. I will show you how easy it is to start applying them in your everyday life.

### *Using the Gunas in Daily Life*

We are constantly affected by changes of the gunas. Among the most important principles of working with these qualities in Ayurvedic treatment as well as daily life are the principles of *like increases like* and *opposites balance.*

**Like Increases Like.** The idea behind like increases like (*samanya*, "similarity") is that, for example, on a cold windy day, automatically in our body the cold, rough, and mobile qualities will be increased, maybe in the form of anxiety, feeling ungrounded, dry skin, or just feeling cold. Similarly, eating a bowl of spicy curry will increase the hot, sharp qualities in our body and mind, manifesting perhaps as sweating, rashes, diarrhea, or irritability. Consuming a bag of oily peanuts will increase the oily quality in our body, maybe manifesting as heaviness, skin breakouts (spots or acne), or slight nausea.

**Opposites Balance.** When an imbalance has manifested, successful treatment simply requires using the opposite qualities (*vishesha*, "dissimilarity"). For example, if there is too much heat (fire) as hot and sharp qualities in our body, we can use cooling drinks, such as coconut water or cucumber water, or a swim in a cool lake to balance this hot quality. If we are consuming ice cream in winter, we can add heating and digestive spices, such as cinnamon or ginger, to counteract the cold, mucous-forming properties of the ice cream. Ayurvedic treatment—no matter if through herbs, massage, diet, or lifestyle—consists to a large extent of identifying which qualities are imbalanced in a person and simply applying the opposites in therapy.

Simple, right? Using these two principles—along with awareness, self-observation, and attunement to body—you can be your own alchemist and influence your physical health and mental well-being tremendously.

## Holy Trinity: Flow (Vata), Transformation (Pitta), and Regeneration (Kapha)

I am only half joking when I call the three doshas, or bioenergies, in Ayurveda the "holy trinity." Trinity is a fundamental concept in Vedic thought. Those of you familiar with Hindu religion and mythology know the three main gods of Hinduism: Brahma (the Creator), Vishnu (the Maintainer), and Shiva (the Destroyer). These gods are symbolic representations of the three aspects of energy that make up the entire universe: creation, maintenance, and destruction. In other words, every event, action, or process has a beginning (Brahma), a duration (Vishnu), and an ending (Shiva).

Before the skeptic in you dismisses this as just a mythological story from India, I invite you to look at the holy trinity through the lens of biology: Shiva is nothing but catabolic energy (Vata); Vishnu, metabolic energy (Pitta); and Brahma, anabolic energy (Kapha). In physics we would call them kinetic energy (Vata), thermal energy (Pitta), and potential energy (Kapha). In computer language, data input/output (Vata), data processing (Pitta), and data storage (Kapha).

Because macro equals micro, this trinity in our body is represented by the three doshas or bioenergies: Vata represents movement and flow; Pitta represents transformation; and Kapha represents regeneration. You will see that the doshas are the organizing principles of the elements in the body and, as such, are responsible for all our physiological and psychological processes. If the elements are musical notes, then the doshas are the symphony.

### *Vata (Ether/Air)*

Derived from the Sanskrit root *vah* (vehicle; to carry, to move), Vata dosha is a combination of the space or ether and air elements. As the principle of mobility, Vata regulates all activity in the body, both mental and physiological. It governs the body's movement and communication, such as peristalsis in the intestines, breathing through the lungs, beating of the heart, movement of limbs, and the flow of thoughts and emotions. The colon is Vata's primary home; it is also present in the brain and nervous system (firing of neurons); heart (beating) and lungs (inhalation and exhalation); and the pelvic region (elimination of urine, gas, and feces; menstruation, childbirth, and ejaculation).

In the body, Vata is in charge of our vital energy—prana or qi. As such, it is often called the "king" of doshas. It is the only dosha that moves actively and can push the other two out of balance. This is why the Ayurvedic classical texts state that most diseases are at root related to an imbalance in Vata dosha.[2]

When in balance, Vata promotes creativity, flexibility, lightness, and joy. Out of balance, it produces fear, nervousness, anxiety, and shakiness. Since the qualities of Vata are dry, light, cold, rough, subtle, mobile, and clear, anything that possesses these qualities has the potential to aggravate Vata in the body. Some of these instigators are natural, such as the seasons; others are due to improper use of food, lifestyle, and exercise.

## What Pushes Vata Out of Balance?

### Natural Daily and Seasonal Cycles

- Whenever there is transition or change, the mobile quality of Vata gets triggered. That is why, during the hours before and around dawn (2 a.m.–6 a.m.) and dusk (2 p.m.–6 p.m.), when night changes into day and vice versa, Vata is naturally increased.
- When the long, hot summer days give way to cold and dryness in fall and early winter (October–January), the cold and dry qualities naturally increase in the environment and our bodies; the same happens throughout the year on cold and windy days.

### Diet

- Dry foods such as crackers, dried fruits, or dried lentils and beans increase Vata's dry and rough qualities.
- Pungent (chili), bitter (coffee, turmeric), and overly astringent (green banana, pomegranates, turmeric) tastes aggravate Vata's dry, rough, and light qualities.
- Iced drinks, cold foods, and raw foods aggravate Vata's cold and rough qualities.
- Skipping meals, insufficient food intake, or dieting increase Vata's light quality.

#### Lifestyle

- Staying up late, not sleeping enough, and overworking increase Vata's light and mobile qualities.
- Multitasking, overstimulation, and traveling increase Vata's mobile quality.
- Stress, fear, and anxiety increase Vata's cold, clear, mobile, and subtle qualities.

### How Do We Know When Vata Is Out of Balance?

Our bodies give us straightforward clues when Vata is imbalanced. We just must learn to listen. When you experience one of the following symptoms due to one or several of Vata's gunas (qualities) being elevated, you know you need to check your Vata.

- Gas, bloating, cramping (cold and rough)
- Constipation (dry and rough)
- Weight and/or muscle loss (light and subtle)
- Feeling "tired but wired"—a hyper state paired with exhaustion (mobile, clear, and light)
- Feeling stressed and overwhelmed (mobile)
- Experiencing dry eyes, skin, hair, and/or brittle nails (dry and rough)
- Cracking, popping joints (dry and rough)
- Having trouble sleeping (clear, light, and mobile)
- Feeling overly anxious, worried, and fearful (clear, light, mobile, and subtle)

### How Do We Balance Elevated Vata?

Once we learn to pay attention to the warning signs of Vata imbalance, we can easily take measures to remedy it by applying the opposite gunas (qualities) for balance. Remember, two of the fundamental tenets of Ayurveda are that like increases like and opposites balance. So, we balance Vata dosha by applying the opposite qualities: warm, moist, heavy, smooth, gross, static, and cloudy.

Vata is mainly cold, light, and dry. So, the easiest way to counter that with your diet is to stick for a while to warm, cooked, and slightly oily and moist foods. Think soups, stews, or cooked oatmeal.

If your mobile quality has been excessively triggered (welcome to modern life!), then creating periods of rest and stability through routine and regularity is vital. This can be as simple as regular meal, bed, and wake-up times; or a yoga or meditation practice that emphasizes stillness and calm (think yin or restorative yoga versus Ashtanga or high-intensity interval training [HIIT]).

If the dry, light, and/or cold qualities are aggravated (such as in fall or when you have a lot of airplane travel), then a regular self-massage with warm sesame oil works wonders.

During times of seasonal change or if you tend to have cold hands or feet, you can easily enhance circulation and digestion by drinking a warm tea of fresh ginger, cardamom, and cinnamon.

### *Pitta (Fire/Water)*

Based on the Sanskrit root *tap* (to heat, shine, burn), Pitta dosha is composed of the fire and water elements. Just like fire transforms everything it encounters, Pitta governs all transformation in the body and mind. In the body, it is responsible for all biochemical processes such as the digestion, absorption, and assimilation of food. It is present as hydrochloric acid, digestive enzymes, heat regulation, and the hormonal system. In the mind, Pitta is responsible for the digestion of thoughts; and in the heart, the transformation and processing of emotions. The small intestine (enzymes, bile) is Pitta's primary seat; secondarily, the brain and nervous system (neurotransmitters), liver (enzymes), spleen (immunity), skin (melanin), eyes (vision), and blood (red blood cells). Pitta combines the qualities of fire and water: hot, sharp, light, liquid, mobile, and oily. When Pitta is in balance, it promotes healthy appetite and vitality, warmth, luster to the skin, clear vision, intelligence, and understanding. Out of balance, it can cause frustration, anger, hatred, and jealousy, as well as general inflammation in the body.

Since Pitta's qualities are hot, sharp, light, liquid, spreading, and oily, anything that possesses these qualities has the potential to aggravate it.

## What Pushes Pitta Out of Balance?

### Natural Daily and Seasonal Cycles

- When the sun (or moon) is at its peak—midday (10 a.m.–2 p.m.) and midnight (10 p.m.–2 a.m.)—Pitta's hot, sharp, and light qualities naturally aggravate.
- During the hot summer months (June–September), Pitta's hot and sharp qualities naturally aggravate.

### Diet

- Hot, spicy, oily, or fried foods aggravate Pitta's hot, sharp, and oily qualities.
- Overly sour (citrus, tomato, vinegar), salty (pickles), and pungent (chili) tastes aggravate Pitta's hot, sharp qualities.
- Coffee, alcohol, and cigarettes are all stimulating and heating and aggravate Pitta's hot and sharp qualities.

### Lifestyle

- Prolonged fasting aggravates Pitta's light quality.
- Prolonged intense exercise aggravates Pitta's hot, sharp, and light qualities.
- Sunbathing aggravates Pitta's hot quality.
- Aggression, ambition, and competition all aggravate Pitta's hot and sharp qualities.

## How Do We Know When Pitta Is Out of Balance?

Again, our bodies give us straightforward clues when Pitta is imbalanced. When Pitta is aggravated, you may experience one or more of the following:

- Heartburn, acidity, reflux (sharp and hot)
- Loose stools or diarrhea (liquid and spreading)
- Excessive sweating (hot and liquid)

- Fatigue, dizziness, vertigo (light)
- Skin rashes, redness (hot and spreading)
- Inflammation, ulceration, infection (hot, sharp, and spreading)
- Irritability, anger, and impatience (hot and sharp)

### How Do We Balance Elevated Pitta?

Once we learn to pay attention to the warning signs of Pitta imbalance, we can easily take measures to remedy it by applying the opposite gunas (qualities) for balance. So, we balance Pitta dosha by applying the following qualities: cool, soft, heavy, dry, and static.

Using food to balance an overheated Pitta system, you would avoid spices, fried or fermented foods, and alcohol. Instead, you may prefer only small amounts of cooling oils such as ghee or coconut oil; and cooling, nonspicy foods such as cucumbers, mung beans, and fresh juicy summer fruits such as melon, peaches, and watermelon. During Pitta peaks in nature, eat plenty of fresh greens, nettles, and other liver-cleansing foods, as well as cooling and hydrating foods such as cucumbers and melons.

During summer, shift your exercise routine to the cooler part of the day and alternate intense workouts with cooling practices such as swimming or yin yoga. Practice more cooling breathing exercises such as *chandra bhedana* (moon breathing). Especially during the hot summer months, drinking a cooling tea of mint, rose, and licorice helps to replenish lost fluids.

### *Kapha (Earth/Water)*

Based on the Sanskrit roots *ka* (water) and *pha* (to flourish), Kapha dosha is a combination of the earth and water elements. In the body and mind, it governs all structure and stability, as well as lubrication and protection. Kapha is the glue that holds our cells together, lubricates our joints, moisturizes our skin, and helps to heal wounds. It is located mainly in the stomach (protective mucous lining); secondarily in the pancreas, brain, spinal cord (white matter; cerebrospinal fluid), kidneys, joints (synovial fluid), oral cavity (saliva), throat and sinuses (mucous lining), and breast tissue (fat, lymph). When Kapha is in balance, it expresses in love, calmness, and forgiveness, as well as immunity, strength, and stamina. Kapha out of balance tends toward depression, attachment, possessiveness, and greed. Physically, there can be excess weight, water retention, and congestion or mucous.

Since Kapha's qualities are heavy, dull, cold, moist/oily, liquid, slimy, dense, soft, static, sticky, and gross, anything that possesses these qualities has the potential to aggravate it.

## What Pushes Kapha Out of Balance?

### Natural Daily and Seasonal Cycles

- Early morning (6 a.m.–10 p.m.) and evening (6 p.m.–10 p.m.) is usually when the air is dampest and heaviest and the cold, heavy, and moist qualities of Kapha increase.
- In late winter and spring (February–May), as the snow starts to melt, Kapha's heavy, moist, and liquid qualities are aggravated.
- On cold, cloudy, or rainy days throughout the year, Kapha's heavy, cold, cloudy, and wet qualities are naturally aggravated.

### Diet

- Cold foods and drinks aggravate Kapha's cold, static qualities.
- Heavy, fatty foods aggravate Kapha's oily and heavy qualities.
- Large meals (overeating) aggravate Kapha's heavy quality.
- Sweet, sour, salty tastes aggravate Kapha's heavy, moist, and liquid qualities.
- Dairy products (cream, cheese, milk, yogurt) aggravate Kapha's oily, sticky, slimy, heavy qualities.

### Lifestyle

- Excessive sleep and daytime napping aggravate Kapha's heavy and static qualities.
- Lack of movement aggravates Kapha's heavy and static qualities.
- Attachment, clinging, and hoarding aggravate Kapha's heavy, sticky, static qualities.

### Symptoms of Kapha Aggravation

- Low appetite and chronic indigestion (heavy, cold, slow)
- Overweight and/or slow metabolism (heavy, cold, slow)
- Cold, cough, and congestion (cold, sticky, cloudy)
- Heaviness, lethargy, and foggy mind (heavy, slow, dull)
- Benign growths such as fibroids, cysts, lipomas (hard, sticky, heavy)
- Edema (moist, dull, static)

## How Do We Balance Elevated Kapha?

Once we learn to pay attention to the warning signs of Kapha imbalance, we can easily take measures to remedy it by applying the opposite gunas (qualities) for balance. So, we balance Kapha dosha by applying the following qualities: light, sharp, hot, dry, rough, hard, mobile, clear, and subtle.

When Kapha dosha is aggravated, it is vital to avoid all mucous-producing foods such as cheese, ice cream, milk, and yogurt—dairy in general has cold, heavy, sticky, and slimy qualities. Also avoid excessive carbohydrates, especially sugar and desserts. Instead, favor foods that are light, warm, and stimulating.

Since Kapha is heavy and static, movement and activity are key. People with significant amounts of Kapha in their constitution or an imbalance usually feel more energetic after movement and more lethargic after rest. So, stimulation, activity, and change are key!

To boost the sluggish metabolism and counter cold and stagnation in the body, cardio exercise, regular sauna, and spicy teas made by boiling ginger, cinnamon, and a pinch of clove help to increase heat and improve circulation.

# 3

## Your Potential

The Matrix of Your Body

### Discover Yourself Through the Lens of Ayurveda

We have seen that the three bioenergies (doshas) are continuously subject to change, influenced by environmental factors such as climate, food, and lifestyle. What does not change, however, is your unique, bio-individual constitution. Each person's combination and proportions of the elements and doshas are determined at the time of conception by the genetics, diet, lifestyle, and emotions of the parents. This is called *prakriti*, or your unique mind-body type. Your prakriti never changes. I like to call it your blueprint, your potential, your individual song in the symphony of life.

Usually people have one or two energies, or doshas, that are predominant in their constitution. But not everybody with the same body type is alike. Remember that the different qualities (*gunas*) of a dosha might express differently in everyone—for example, one Vata person might express more cold quality; another Vata person, more light or dry qualities.

### Why Most Dosha Tests Fail

These days, there is much confusion about constitutions, not the least because most online dosha quizzes do not distinguish between constitution (*prakriti*) and imbalance (*vikriti*). People in the West generally are obsessed with their "type," while doctors in India could not care less. Understandably, doctors are generally focused on treating the imbalance in a person because it is the pathology that is crucial for disease and treatment. People in the West often overly identify and lock themselves into their dosha or constitution; as a result, they narrow their diet and lifestyle to that without considering the balanced expression and nature of a dosha and the ever-changing dance that happens in our bodies in sync with the rhythms of our environment. Instead of learning to flow with life, they become overly rigid, stagnant, and ultimately imbalanced.

### *The Danger of Overidentifying with a State of Imbalance Dosha Assessment*

An overidentification with an imbalanced state happens mainly because constitutional assessments and profiling are already pathologized. For example, it is commonly accepted that Vata constitutions are cold; they have dry skin, frequent bloating and constipation, and are generally hyperactive and anxious. So, should Vatas only eat warm soups and porridge and become couch potatoes? Of course not. Movement, change, and excitement are in the very nature of Vata, so they need to be properly expressed and cultivated in a balanced way. To be clear, a balanced Vata is not always cold and does not have overly dry skin, nor are they continuously bloated, constipated, or a nervous wreck. These are all signs of a Vata imbalance. To repeat: Your unique body type is different from your current body, emotional state, your acquired personality or survival strategies, and your diseases. Those are all factors that continuously change during your lifetime.

## A Revolutionary New Approach to Determining Your Body Type (*Prakriti*)

In this light, I propose that prakriti should be strictly assessed based on *unchanging* features, such as:

- The shape (bone structure) of your body
- The shape of your face
- The shape of your hands
- Your overall metabolic strength
- Your general temperament
- Your general stress response (physical/mental)

## Somatotyping Body Shapes

Interestingly, there is a direct correspondence between Ayurveda's tridosha framework and the science of somatotyping, developed by the American psychologist William H. Sheldon in the 1940s. Somatotyping is a way to assess body type and shape, and analyze individual physical characteristics, health risks, and potential. Sheldon classified people into three general body types based primarily on their body shape: ectomorphic, mesomorphic, and endomorphic. He created these terms borrowing from the three germ layers of embryonic development: the endoderm, which develops into the digestive tract; the mesoderm, which becomes muscle, heart, and blood vessels; and the ectoderm, which forms the skin and nervous system. According to this Western classification system:

Ectomorphs (Vata) are thin and long-limbed with a delicate build.
Mesomorphs (Pitta) are strong and muscular with a medium build.
Endomorphs (Kapha) are soft and round or square with a heavy build.

Each body type has its own unique set of physical characteristics and predispositions. *Ectomorphs* are closely linked to skin, membranes, and the nervous system; Vata governs sensing and nervous activity. *Mesomorphs* are linked to muscle, heart, and blood vessels; the blood is the only tissue in the body related to Pitta. *Endomorphs* are linked to the digestive tract; digestion is all about anabolic activity—using food for energy and to build tissue—such as Kapha.

The somatotyping categories, the doshas, and the elements inform each other to help clarify our body type profile. Vata types are ectomorphs. Just like the nature of wind, their core biological blueprint is *catabolic*, related to movement and a resulting breakdown of tissues. Challenge points are depletion, degeneration, and nervous system overwhelm. Pitta types are mesomorphs. Just like the nature of fire, their core biological blueprint is *metabolic*, related to transformation and digestion. Challenge points are acidity and inflammation. Kapha types are endomorphs. Just like the nature of water, their core biological blueprint is *anabolic*, related to lubrication, protection, and regeneration. Challenge points are excess weight, sluggishness, and congestion. If you were to draw yourself in terms of overall bone structure and body composition, a Vata person would be a long or short line; a Pitta person, a pointed triangle; and a Kapha person, a circle/oval or square/rectangle.

## Constitution as Potential

Think about your constitution not as a fixed label but a potentiality, and life as a journey toward fulfilling that potential so you can contribute your unique gift to the world. This is why, in the coming chapter, I will start talking about the three doshas in their constitutional expressions as Movers (Vata, or V), Transformers (Pitta, or P), and Regenerators (Kapha, or K). I use these terms to help you avoid falling into pathologizing too easily and to give you a much better sense of the essence and positive expression of each constitutional type.

## What Am I? Assessing Your Ayurvedic Metabolic Blueprint (*Prakriti*)

Place a checkmark next to the answer that best reflects your *general* tendencies throughout life and *not* the way you are now.

1. What is the shape or frame of your body (when healthy or compared to family members, ethnic group)?
   - ☐ Rectangular, with heavy bones and/or round, curvaceous (K)
   - ☐ Triangular and muscular (P)
   - ☐ Petite and light bones or very tall and slender (V)

2. What is the shape of your face?
   - ☐ Rectangular, square, and/or round (K)
   - ☐ Triangular, heart-shaped, with prominent bones (jaw, cheekbones) and tapering chin (P)
   - ☐ Oblong, narrow, asymmetrical (V)

3. What is the shape of your hands?
   - ☐ Large and solid or soft hand (K)
   - ☐ Medium with muscular, firm grip (P)
   - ☐ Tiny hands or long, slender fingers (V)

4. How is your skin and complexion?
   - ☐ Thicker; moist, well lubricated (K)
   - ☐ Fair and sensitive; reactive; oily (P)
   - ☐ Darker; often dry and rough (V)

5. What best describes your temperament?
   - ☐ Methodical and caring: detail-oriented, patient, tolerant, gentle (K)
   - ☐ Analytical: goal-oriented, competitive, challenge-driven (P)
   - ☐ Creative and enthusiastic: open-minded, easygoing, adaptable (V)

6. How about your mental activity?
   - ☐ You have a calm and steady mind. (K)
   - ☐ You have sharp intellect. (P)
   - ☐ You have a quick and restless mind. (V)

7. How is your concentration and focus?
   - ☐ Methodical and detailed; slow learner but great long-term memory and focus (K)
   - ☐ Great ability to concentrate and focus; sharp intellect (P)
   - ☐ Fast learner but memory and focus often short term; tendency toward attention deficit disorder (ADD) or attention deficit hyperactivity disorder (ADHD) (V)

8. In general, your appetite is:
   - ☐ Steady—you tend to feel full for a while after meals and can easily skip meals if needed, but you love to eat and are often an emotional eater. (K)

- ☐ Strong—you don't like to skip meals and can get irritable if you eat late or skip meals. (P)
- ☐ Inconsistent—your appetite fluctuates, and you tend to nibble and need to eat more frequently; when busy, you often forget to eat and can get hypoglycemic. (V)

9. Your lifelong tendency with weight has been:
   - ☐ You have a slow metabolism and gain weight easily; it is difficult for you to lose weight. (K)
   - ☐ You can gain or lose weight easily, depending on what you focus on. (P)
   - ☐ You don't gain weight easily and sometimes even have trouble keeping it on. (V)

10. Which type of weather do you generally prefer and feel best in?
    - ☐ Warm and dry (K)
    - ☐ Cool and mild (P)
    - ☐ Warm and moist (V)

11. Off-balance physically, you most frequently experience:
    - ☐ Heaviness, sluggishness, weight gain, congestion, or mucous (K)
    - ☐ Inflammation, overheating and sweating, skin rashes, or acidity (P)
    - ☐ Hyperactivity, nervousness, insomnia, loss of appetite, exhaustion (V)

12. What is your general emotional stress response?
    - ☐ Freeze: stubborn, rigid, paralyzed, depressed, lethargic (K)
    - ☐ Fight: frustrated, angry, impatient, irritable (P)
    - ☐ Flight: anxious, nervous, scattered, overwhelmed (V)

Total: K______ P______ V______

Please count how many checkmarks you marked in each category: Vata (V), Pitta (P), Kapha (K). The highest score is your main constitutional type. If you have a close second score, you are a dual doshic type.

V= Vata = MOVER

P = Pitta = TRANSFORMER

K = Kapha = REGENERATOR

## Discover Your Unique Skills, Gifts, and Assets

Even though there are as many constitutional types as there are people on the planet, for simplicity's sake, we can divide people into seven basic constitutional types:

1. Vata (Movers)
2. Pitta (Transformers)
3. Kapha (Regenerators)
4. Vata-Pitta/Pitta-Vata (Mover-Transformers)
5. Pitta-Kapha/Kapha-Pitta (Regenerator-Transformers)
6. Vata-Kapha/Kapha-Vata (Mover-Regenerators)
7. Vata-Pitta-Kapha (Mover-Transformer-Regenerators)

Knowledge is power. Learning what your somato- or body type is can give you an excellent road map to navigate the challenges and stress that come with being a human in this world.

### *Stress Occurs When Demand Outweighs Skill*

Remember that stress does not occur just because our life is busy or we do too much. Stress occurs simply when demand outweighs skill. If a Mover (Vata) is working in a nine-to-five office job as an accountant crunching numbers, with no room for creative expression and unconventional thinking, at some point their system will crack. Why? Because stability, precision, analysis, and methodological thinking are not their forte. They are spending energy that is not coming naturally to them, and they are suppressing their innate need for change, creativity, stimulation, and interaction. Similarly, a Transformer (Pitta) who is stuck in a relationship where passion and intimacy are gone and conversations focus on the kids' school activities will ultimately become sick because their needs for passion, challenge, intellectual exchange, and adventurous companionship are not met. Health, balance, and vitality are actually first and foremost about finding your constitution's gift, skill set, and potential. Once you find your mojo, you groove instead of pushing uphill.

## Are You a Mover (Vata)?

Movers are naturally born:

Creatives
Trendsetters
Communicators
Connecters
Dreamers
Thinkers

Given their elemental composition of space and air, Movers' nature is that of flow. They are flexible and adaptable, adjusting easily to changing plans, new environments, and unexpected twists and turns. Easygoing, enthusiastic, and bright, Movers are contagiously joyful creatures. When they enter a room, the party begins.

### *Fast and Furious*

Due to the mobile quality of air, Movers are fast and agile. They learn fast, easily grasp new concepts (but also forget easily), and love multitasking and juggling diverse tasks or projects at once. Quick-minded, spontaneous, creative, and full of new ideas, Movers can easily make things happen. Movers are also intuitive sensers; they sense trends often long before they become mainstream. Movers dream big—they can envision and make things happen. Start-ups almost always have Movers on their team. Movers are true artists and philosophers at heart: sensitive, creative, eccentric, and high-strung. Social butterflies and loners at the same time, Movers resist predictability and regularity.

### *Thinking Out of the Box*

Movers are natural communicators and often choose creative professions in the expressive arts (theater, painting, writing), journalism, marketing, advertising, or public relations. If their job involves traveling and adventure, they love it even more. Movers are adaptable, able to think "out of the box," and willing to walk the untrodden paths. This is also true regarding their spiritual journeys. Movers have a keen interest in breaking old patterns, self-developing, and evolving. It is not uncommon for Movers to be attracted to various spiritual or religious traditions and mix them into a religion of their own. Due to the light and subtle quality of the space and air element, Movers are born meditators, yet often their restless mind and body as well as general hyperactivity prevent them from sitting still and sticking to a regular practice.

### *Relationships: Warm, Open, and Joyful*

Movers bring an open mind, joy, curiosity, and adventure to relationships. Mover relationships do not run the risk of getting stuck in a rut. Movers are good communicators; they can express feelings and needs easily and openly. Due to the mobile quality, Movers do not hold on to grudges and can easily let go of disagreements or arguments. They are also radically open to change and evolution—in themselves and their partners. As touch is the sense connected to the air element, Movers love touching and being touched as a gesture of affection.

### *Physical Makeup: Lean, Agile, and Energetic*

- **Body frame and face:** Due to their elemental composition (air and ether), Movers either have a long and lanky skeletal frame or are tiny and petite. Their shoulders and hips are narrow, and their weight is usually low, often due to a fast metabolism, undereating, and general hyperactivity. Movers have light or weak bones and joints that are prone to cracking and popping. Hands and feet are either long and narrow with bony fingers, or tiny. Facial features are chiseled, angular, and irregular, with eyes that are small and set deep.

- **Skin and hair:** Movers' skin tone is usually on the darker side, and they tan easily. Their skin is on the thin and dry side and will usually show early signs of aging and wrinkles. Their hair is also often dry, rough, and frizzy. Cold in nature, Movers usually love heat and warm climates. Their health is usually much better during the summer months and in humid or tropical climates.
- **Digestion and metabolism:** Sensitive as they are, Movers' digestion can be variable, and often their eyes are bigger than their stomachs. After meals—especially when they've eaten too fast—they can experience gas and bloating, as well as dry stools and irregular elimination. If their mind is busy and they are excited, Movers can easily forget to eat, or they just nibble and skip proper meals. But out of all types, they do best with scheduled meals.
- **Energy, stamina, sleep:** Movers' bodies and minds are light and agile, and they thrive on action and movement. They are high-energy people but often lack stamina and resources to support their speed. Movers are light sleepers. With their active minds, they usually have a hard time falling asleep, and they can wake up frequently at night, especially when disturbed by sounds or noise. They dream a lot—often intense, active dreams involving motion, flying, or being chased. Movers tend to sleep fewer hours than most—six to seven, on average—but their bodies and minds require more sleep than other constitutions. In the stillness of sleep, Movers' active and catabolic nature is countered, nourished, and restored. Movers are morning people. They have no problem waking up early and alert, ready to jump out of bed immediately and start the day. On the other hand, toward the end of the day, Movers' energy drops; they run out of steam and usually are ready to go to bed early.

## Are You a Transformer (Pitta)?

Transformers are natural:

Thinkers
Leaders
Activists
Problem-solvers
Teachers
Doers
Challengers

The biggest virtue of Transformers is their courage. They are picture-book type A personalities: determined, goal-oriented, sharp-minded, and strong-willed.

### *Thriving on Challenge*

Transformers stand up for what they believe in and do not shy away from confrontation and challenge. In fact, Transformers thrive on challenge. They are natural leaders and planners, and they have a dominant personality. While competitive and ambitious, they stick to values and principles as well as fair play. Transformers are intelligent, discerning, and articulate. They have a great capacity for concentration, research, and analysis. They love knowledge and intellectual stimulation and have a great visual learning capacity. Often they choose professions such as politics, trading, management, research, and teaching.

### *Natural Skeptics*

Usually skeptics by nature, Transformers have an ambivalent relationship with faith and do not easily surrender to any religion or belief system. They have an innate need to understand, comprehend, and make sense, so belief and faith are not their forte.

### *Relationships: Passionate and Intense*

Having the fire element as a constitutional characteristic, Transformers need a relationship that is passionate and sexually fulfilling. They thrive on both physical and intellectual connections that are based on clear communication and intellectual stimulation. Natural-born leaders, Transformers also like to take the lead in their intimate relationships when it comes to providing for family, planning, organizing, and making decisions.

### *Physical Makeup: Athletic, Muscular, and Hot-Blooded*

- **Body frame and face:** Transformers are medium build and athletic, with well-developed muscles and a solid bone structure. Their bodies are usually well-balanced and proportionate, and their metabolism is strong. Their face is heart-shaped, often with sharp facial features such as a pointed nose or a tapered chin.
- **Skin and hair:** Transformers have fair and sensitive skin, with moles and a pinkish complexion. They are sensitive to the sun, prone to rashes and skin allergies, and become red easily (when blushing or with strenuous exercise). Their hair is thin, fine, and straight, often copper or a light color. Out of all constitutions, Transformers tend to early onset of gray hair as well as early balding. Their eyes are medium in size, light in color (blue, green, or gray) and can be piercing and intense.
- **Digestion and metabolism:** Transformers have a strong appetite and metabolism, and their weight tends to be steady, even though they can gain and lose weight easily depending on activities and lifestyle. They do not like skipping meals, are a pain to be around when hangry (hungry + angry), and usually desire large quantities of food and fluids. Out of balance, their digestion tends toward loose stools and diarrhea as well as reflux and heartburn. Transformers generally feel warm and overheat or sweat easily, especially when exercising or moving. As a result, Transformers do much better in cooler seasons and climates.
- **Energy, stamina, and sleep:** Transformers usually have good energy and stamina and a strong will and determination to pull things through. But due to their ambitious and competitive nature, they can at times get carried away and push themselves over the edge, ignoring the needs and limits of their bodies and

minds. Transformers sleep easily and wake up alert. However, they tend to stay up late and often get a second wind after 10 p.m. (Pitta time), when they will spend too much time following their interests, passions, or projects. Usually Transformers remember their dreams well, which are often passionate, intense, and involve heat or light, as well as chasing and control.

## Are You a Regenerator (Kapha)?

Regenerators are natural:

Carers
Nourishers
Listeners
Supporters
Preservers
Managers
Collectors

The biggest assets of Regenerators are their patience, care, and compassion. Regenerator types are immensely pleasant to be around. They are cheerful, sweet, easygoing, good-natured, calm, patient, and tolerant. They have very stable personalities and love security. Family, close friends, and home are their comfort zones.

### *Playing It Safe*

Regenerators like to play it safe. They do not easily take risks, and they take their sweet time making decisions, weighing all the options back and forth. However, unlike Movers, once Regenerators decide, they are committed and dedicated for life. While they are slow learners, Regenerators have excellent long-term memory and are very structured and methodical. Regarding faith and religion, they can be strong believers, and they have a stable, unwavering faith that comes naturally. They do not experiment or shop around, often sticking to the religious belief they were brought up with.

### *Relationships: Stable, Dedicated, and Loyal*

Regenerators have rock-solid, stable personalities and are not easily thrown off-balance. They are caring and nurturing beings, and as a result, their relationships usually are steady and long-term. They do not feel much need to go out and conquer the world but instead are happy to create nourishing and intimate relationships with loved ones at home. Regenerators love to care for others and nurture, whether it is for partners, children, friends, plants, animals, or projects. They are reliable, trustworthy, dedicated, and loyal. They seek relationships that give them comfort through connection and commitment while being easeful and free of drama.

### *Physical Makeup*

- **Body frame and face:** Due to their elemental composition (earth and water), Regenerators are heavyset: They have a round or square face, a broad body frame, large hips, and round shoulders. Often with strong bones and large, square hands and feet, Regenerators enjoy great strength, stability, and stamina.
- **Skin and hair:** Regenerators have strong teeth, as well as smooth, thick, and oily skin. They usually age well and often do not show any sign of wrinkles until later in life. Their hair is lush, thick, and often wavy, and their eyes big and beautiful.
- **Digestion and metabolism:** Regenerators have a passion for food and usually enjoy cooking and eating immensely. They often have an emotional rather than an actual appetite and tend toward sluggishness and weight gain. While they love food and eating, Regenerators are slow burners and can easily skip meals without a drop in energy. On the contrary, they feel great when eating less or fasting, and despite their bigger build, they do not require large amounts of food. Regenerators' bowels are usually well lubricated and their stool naturally well-formed and bulky.
- **Energy, stamina, and sleep:** Out of all constitutions, Regenerators have the greatest stamina and endurance (both physically and emotionally), which often is greatly underutilized because they love chilling, playing it safe, and being cozy and comfortable.

However, if they are committed to being active, they have a strong and sturdy constitution and are blessed with good health and a long life. Even though Regenerators actually thrive on less sleep (five to six hours is usually enough for them), due to the heavy quality of earth and water, they love sleeping and have a hard time getting out of bed in the morning, especially if they sleep well into Kapha time (6 a.m.–10 a.m.). They sleep deeply and have calm and uneventful dreams, sometimes with a romantic twist.

## Are You a Combination (Dual- or Tri-doshic)?

While some people are singular expressions and embodiment of one dosha, most people tend to be a combination of two, where one dosha predominates and the other is secondary. In this case, many of the characteristics of the predominant dosha will feature along with some traits of the secondary.

## Mover-Transformers (Vata-Pitta)

A person who exhibits both Mover and Transformer qualities cannot tolerate excessive heat or cold. They like milder climates; they have a strong appetite but a changing digestion and variable elimination. Mover-Transformers are usually lean with good muscles and a strong metabolism. They also have an enthusiastic, curious, and sharp mind and a captivating and charismatic personality.

### *Smart and Sassy*

Mover-Transformers are generally smart, sassy, fun, and full of ideas. They love to learn, they're quick thinkers, and they're creative problem-solvers. Mover-Transformers are trendsetters, fire starters, and leaders with vision. They dream, set goals, and go for it. They are natural

Creative thinkers
Passionate problem-solvers
Visionary leaders

Inspiring teachers
Transformational dreamers

*Relationships: Curious and Passionate*

Mover-Transformers also bring curiosity, passion, excitement, and adventure to their relationships. They thrive on shared goals, interests, and life vision with their partner. Clear communication and intellectual stimulation is vital for them. Physically they thrive on affection, touch, seduction, and passion.

*Physical Makeup: Lean and Muscular*

- **Body frame and face:** Mover-Transformers have a light-to-medium bone structure and narrow shoulders and hips. Their musculature is lean and muscular, and their weight generally stable but on the lower end. The shape of their face is oval and can be irregular, with a tapered chin and rather sharp and angular features.
- **Skin and hair:** The skin is darker than typical Transformer skin yet sensitive and often a combination type. Similarly, the hair also can be fine and oily or dry. Mover-Transformers prefer warm but mild climates and a moderate amount of sun.
- **Digestion and metabolism:** Mover-Transformers usually have a strong appetite but variable digestion. Their metabolism is high, and they feel best with two to three (larger) meals daily to supply their fast metabolic needs. To counter digestive imbalances, they need to emphasize eating slowly, preferably in a quiet and calm setting rather than working lunches or eating while multitasking or in a rush.
- **Energy, stamina, and sleep:** Mover-Transformers have a light and agile body, and a smart mind full of curiosity. They are high-energy, full-power people who are comfortable with action, challenge, and change. Mover-Transformer types are light sleepers and generally wake up alert and fresh, ready to greet a new day and tackle their projects. Even though they tend to sleep fewer hours than most, this combo may require more sleep for rest and recuperation.

## Transformer-Regenerators (Pitta-Kapha)

Out of all constitutional types, the Transformer-Regenerator combination is best suited for today's changeable, chaotic world. This dual type has the stability of Regenerators paired with the fire of Transformers. Usually they enjoy good health and a balanced personality. Because both doshas share the oily and moist qualities, this combination has naturally soft and smooth skin, well-lubricated joints, and a capacity to relax into unexpected twists and turns.

Transformer-Regenerators are generally stable and grounded, thoughtful and discerning. Their mind is calm and steady, with good concentration, memory, and articulate speech. Transformer-Regenerators are also extremely hardworking and reliable. They love learning and teaching, and they have a natural capacity for details, analysis, and problem-solving. They are

Methodical thinkers
Compassionate leaders
Protective activists
Detailed problem-solvers
Caring mentors

### *Relationships: Passionate and Caring*

Transformer-Regenerators bring both care and romance to relationships. They are dedicated and loyal, and they like to nourish their family and friends. While they seek connection and commitment, they also need a sense of challenge and adventure to keep their passion alive and to prevent them from getting stuck in a rut.

### *Physical Makeup: Solid and Strong*

- **Body frame and face:** Transformer-Regenerators have a solid body with a sturdy bone structure, well-developed muscles, and usually a few extra pounds. Their face is a blend of Regenerator roundness with Transformer sharper features. Their eyes are likely large and usually warm and captivating.

- **Skin and hair:** Their skin is fair, pinkish, thick, and slightly oily. Their hair is strong and shiny.
- **Digestion and metabolism:** Transformer-Regenerators have a steady appetite and a passion for food. They tend to overindulge in sweets and carbs as well as emotional eating. While their metabolism is sturdy, if overeating, they tend to easily put on weight. Elimination is regular and usually soft and well-formed.
- **Energy, stamina, and sleep:** In general, the balanced combination of earth, water, and fire makes a sturdy and resilient constitution with stable energy, strong immunity, and excellent overall health. Combining the drive of Transformers with the compassion and endurance of Regenerators, this combo makes for great athletes, caring managers, and thoughtful leaders. Transformer-Regenerators' sleep is deep and easeful. They do well with six or seven hours on average. While they may have the capacity to be quite productive late at night, they will suffer heaviness, sluggishness, and weight gain when waking up long after sunrise.

## Mover-Regenerators (Vata-Kapha)

United in their cold quality, people with the mix of Mover and Regenerator energies are sensitive to cold environments and foods. They do best living in warmer climates and focusing on warm and lightly spiced foods. Mover-Regenerators are gentle, humorous, and lovable personalities who do not easily lose their cool.

Mover-Regenerator types have many opposing qualities (heavy-light, dry-oily, static-moving), and that contradiction is usually expressed in their temperament. They can be funny and enthusiastic, yet also gentle and sweet; they are dreamers, yet also detail-oriented; they are creative and analytical but can be speedy and patient. They are

Compassionate communicators
Nourishing connecters
Detailed dreamers
Grounded creatives

Steady thinkers
Eclectic collectors

*Relationships: Joyful and Emotional*

Mover-Regenerators bring joy, ease, and care to relationships. While they need stability and security, they also easily feel stuck in a rut and do well with keeping things unpredictable. Both Mover and Regenerator personalities are sensitive and emotional, which makes Mover-Regenerators exceptionally aware and attuned to their partner's needs and feelings but they are also easily hurt.

*Physical Makeup: Tall and Soft*

- **Body frame and face:** Mover-Regenerators are often tall with a moderate bone structure and a soft body with less defined muscles. Their weight can easily fluctuate. Their face is a blend of Regenerator roundness and Mover length and irregularity. Their eyes are medium in size and lively.
- **Skin and hair:** Both skin and hair are usually moderately thick and well-nourished. Mover-Regenerators share the cold quality, so they tend to feel cold easily and prefer warmer and sunnier climates.
- **Digestion and metabolism:** Lacking the fire element, Mover-Regenerators have a variable digestion, generally low appetite, and sluggish elimination. They do well with two regular meals that are spaced out evenly throughout the day to give their bodies plenty of time to digest.
- **Energy, stamina, and sleep:** In general, Movers can have energy bursts they cannot sustain, while Regenerators have great stamina but tend to be sluggish and lethargic. For this combo, it is important to strike a balance between activity and rest, stimulation and relaxation, change and routine. Mover-Regenerators usually sleep well but do best to go to bed early and wake up before sunrise to avoid the heaviness of Kapha energy.

## Mover-Transformer-Regenerators (Tri-doshic; Equal Vata-Pitta-Kapha)

Tri-doshic constitutions—where all three energetic forces are equal—are blessed with exceptional genes and excellent health. They are not easily thrown off and enjoy strength, immunity, vitality, and long life.

### *The Best of All Worlds*

Mover-Transformer-Regenerators have the best of all worlds. They are sweet and smart; funny and hardworking; courageous and compassionate. This tri-doshic combo is uniquely capable of generating, articulating, and then realizing their visions and dreams. Easygoing and open-minded, Mover-Transformer-Regenerators are not easily thrown off with challenge. They succeed in a fast-paced and chaotic world through their unique combination of drive, creativity, and passion, paired with patience and compassion. They are a sweet mix of

Connecters
Dreamers
Thinkers
Leaders
Problem-solvers
Teachers
Preservers
Managers

### *Blessing and Curse*

I sometimes say the Mover-Transformer-Regenerator combo type is both a blessing and a curse. It's a blessing because it makes for an exceptionally resilient type. It's a curse exactly for that same reason. Tri-doshic constitutions can easily get away with no sleep, overworking, poor nutrition, or large amounts of caffeine and alcohol without noticing the damage these can cause in the long run. With this body type, a serious disease often seems to appear out of the blue in their forties or fifties but in fact surfaced after decades of low-grade, unnoticed imbalances.

### *Relationships: Open-Minded, Caring, and (Com)passionate*

In relationships, Mover-Transformer-Regenerators also have the best of all worlds. They bring curiosity, (com)passion, joy, and ease to relationships. They are supportive, caring, sensitive, and well-attuned to their partner's needs and feelings. Mover-Transformer-Regenerators are good communicators and excellent listeners, open to change and evolving together with their partner. They are also fiercely loyal, generous, and affectionate.

### *Physical Makeup: Well-Proportioned and Strong*

- **Body frame and face:** Mover-Transformer-Regenerators have a well-proportioned frame that is medium in size, with exceptional strength and stamina. Their musculature is well-formed, strong, and slightly round, and their weight is usually stable. Their face may include a combination of Mover angularity, Transformer sharpness, and Regenerator softness and roundness. Eyes are medium in size, bright, and shining.
- **Skin and hair:** Mover-Transformer-Regenerators have soft, hydrated, and lustrous skin and hair. Joints are round, smooth, and well lubricated, and body temperature is neutral, equally comfortable in both hot and cold climactic conditions.
- **Digestion and metabolism:** Mover-Transformer-Regenerators have a steady appetite, and they enjoy food. Their digestive excellence allows them to eat almost anything without discomfort. When they are healthy, their elimination operates like clockwork and their stools are well-formed. Weight is usually balanced, stable, and proportionate.
- **Energy, stamina, and sleep:** With the three doshas equal, Mover-Transformer-Regenerators are sturdy and have excellent overall health, strong immunity, stable energy, and vitality. When in balance, they sleep soundly and wake easily. They require little-

to-moderate amounts of sleep—six hours are usually enough—and wake up easily and refreshed, especially when getting out of bed before sunrise in the morning.

## Summary: Simple but Not Simplistic

The idea of constitutional typing is simple but by no means simplistic or rigid. Each human being is unique, with a mind-body like no other. We are not labels or categories. Remember that just because two people have the same constitution does not mean that the doshas or temperaments express equally in the two. Do not take the constitutional types as stereotypes but rather as guidelines or points of view on some of your innate physical and psycho-emotional tendencies. Your constitution is a foundation on which to build and a potential to be fulfilled. No constitution is better than another, so rather than trying to become someone else, we can try to evolve into the best version of ourselves. We can evolve from a scattered and nervous Mover into an open and creative one; from a controlling and angry Transformer into a courageous and passionate one; and from a lazy and stubborn Regenerator into a compassionate and patient one.

## Your Imbalance or Growth Points (*Vikriti*)

*Vikriti* means "after creation" (*vi*, "after"; *kriti*, "creation"), so your vikriti is everything that happens after you were conceived by your parents. Vikriti is a snapshot of your current physical and mental-emotional state. Remember, along with your assets and skills, your constitution (*prakriti*) also gives you particular tendencies, challenges, and growth points. In a way, yes, your prakriti can predispose you to certain types of imbalances. A Mover type is generally more prone to developing Vata type imbalances than others. But keep in mind that your imbalance can also be radically different from your body type. If a Mover eats a carton of ice cream every night while streaming movies, eventually they will develop mucous, congestion, lethargy, and weight gain (Kapha imbalances).

### *Vikriti Is Always Changeable*

Vikriti includes your current body, acquired personality, emotional state, and diseases. Those are all factors that are subject to change from day to day, season to season, or even in different stages of life. So vikriti is best understood as the doshic tendencies, imbalances, and symptoms that are expressed in the now.

## Mover (Vata) Vikriti: Restless, Hyperactive, and Depleted

Due to their elemental composition (air and ether elements), Movers can easily become restless and hyperactive. Juggling too many balls at once and pressured by FOMO (fear of missing out), they tend to over-exert themselves and then exhaust easily. Sensitive as they are, Movers usually have delicate health and can easily get depleted, burned out, and overwhelmed. With stress, their immune system plummets, and they can be susceptible to (viral) infections such as colds and flu.

### *Digestion and Metabolism: Variable*

Due to the air element, Movers' digestion can become variable, and both appetite and elimination can change easily. Especially when skipping meals, frequently snacking, or eating too fast, Movers can experience gas and bloating. Due to excessive dryness in their systems, they can also easily be constipated, especially when their routines are off or they are traveling. Already fast metabolizers, Movers have a hard time putting on weight or building muscles. Since they can easily forget to eat, their blood sugar drops, leaving them dizzy, hypoglycemic, and low in energy. Movers certainly do best with three regular, warm, and nourishing meals per day.

### *Energy, Stamina, and Sleep: Overcommitted and Overworked*

Movers are hyperactive and love juggling many balls at once. They are passionate and curious yes-sayers. As a result, they tend to be over-committed, overworked, and powered-out. Due to the light quality of the ether and air elements, a Mover's active mind often prevents them from falling asleep easily, and they can wake up frequently at night, especially when disturbed by sounds or noise. Insomnia is not uncommon for imbalanced Movers.

### *Mental-Emotional: Changeable and Anxious*

Movers crave change and tend to easily fall in love (with somebody or something), yet just as fast they lose interest and drop everything. Often they lack persistence and dedication and have difficulty concentrating or completing tasks or sticking to one area of interest. Movers may start learning Spanish one month, move on to dancing tango the next, only then to discover their love for kitesurfing. Nothing is long-lived in the Mover universe. Their challenge is to "stick it out," commit themselves, and persevere. Psychologically, when out of balance, Movers tend toward anxiety, fear, stress, nervousness, and tension. They can feel disconnected, lonely, and ungrounded. Movers are sensitive and high-strung, and with adversities or challenges can become discouraged and give up easily. They generally do well with (group) support and encouragement.

### *Relationships: Serial Daters*

While Movers are spontaneous, warm, easygoing, and fun to be around, commitment is not their forte. Movers can easily feel stuck and stifled, especially in a long-term relationship. They tend to prefer open relationships or resort to being short-term, serial daters, moving from partner to partner like hummingbirds. If they are in a committed relationship, their challenge will be to ground and root with their partner and together explore ways of nourishing their spontaneous, freedom-loving nature.

### *Disease Pattern: Depletion and Degeneration*

A Mover's disease pattern often tends to be stress-related, digestive, or neurological. When overworked, Movers can develop adrenal depletion, burnout, and exhaustion; psychosomatic problems; and digestive issues such as chronic constipation or irritable bowel syndrome (IBS).

If their imbalances progress as they age, Movers are prone to developing degenerative bone diseases such as osteoporosis or arthritis, as well as neurodegenerative disorders such as Parkinson's or multiple sclerosis (MS).

**Shadow and Growth Points**
Superficiality
Fear
Detachment
Disconnection

## Transformer (Pitta) Vikriti

Due to their elemental composition (fire and water), Transformers can overheat, sweat excessively, and develop systemic inflammation. Their body pH will quickly tilt toward acidity, especially with the overconsumption of alcohol, coffee, animal protein, fried foods, or sugar. In the long run, this can lead to an increased risk of (bacterial) infections, decreased energy production in the cells, inflammation, and inability to detoxify heavy metals and other toxic metabolic wastes.

### *Digestion and Metabolism: Heartburn and Acidity*

Even though Transformers have a strong appetite and digestion, if they overindulge in processed, spicy, and fried foods, they can develop heartburn, reflux, and diarrhea. If not corrected, this eventually may lead to gastritis, ulcers, or even inflammatory bowel diseases (IBD) such as Crohn's or ulcerative colitis.

### *Energy, Stamina, and Sleep: Pushing Beyond Limits*

While a Transformer usually has a good supply of energy and stamina, they run the risk of getting carried away and pushing themselves beyond the capacity and limit of their body due to their driven, ambitious, and competitive nature. This eventually can lead to burnout, systemic inflammation, high blood pressure, and/or heart disease.

Transformers love to stay up past midnight, when they get a second wind, feel productive, and work on projects and deadlines. Unfortunately this falls into the period when the transformative energy of the liver is most active (10 p.m.–2 a.m.). During this time, the body detoxifies, clears out wastes, and recalibrates for the following day. If Transformers continuously miss that window, they can get overly inflamed and acidic. As the liver becomes sluggish, they may develop headaches and body stiffness; their skin may become impure, red, and inflamed; and their hormonal balance may be disturbed.

### *Mental-Emotional: Arrogant and Aggressive*

While balanced, Transformers are courageous, committed, and charismatic go-getters. Out of balance, they can be a pain to be around. They become self-centered, controlling, bossy, and arrogant. Discipline and hard work can easily become overambition, overdrive, and perfectionism. Pushing themselves and others over the limit, Transformers end up frustrated, short-tempered, impatient, and overly critical or judgmental (of self and others). They can also slip into narcissistic fanaticism, imposing their likes, beliefs, and behaviors onto everyone around them.

### *Relationships: Critical and Controlling*

In intimate relationships, an imbalanced Transformer can easily turn from a passionate, attentive, and charming lover to being extremely jealous, critical, and dominating. During conflict, a Transformer's shadow side is usually to blame; rarely do they see the fault in themselves. Their standard reaction to conflict is usually "What have you done wrong?" If there is a long history of fighting, hurt, and trauma, they can even resort to cruelty and violence. Their challenge will be to soften irritation and criticism. If they can make space for self-reflection, they will be able to soften the blows and see that "It's my way or the highway" is ultimately alienating them from the people around them.

### *Disease Pattern: Inflammatory*

Transformer disease patterns tend to be inflammatory, due to the excess fire element. They can develop stress-related high blood pressure and heart disease, and they tend toward inflammatory skin diseases such as acne and rosacea, as well as autoimmune conditions such as Crohn's, colitis, lupus, rheumatoid arthritis, or psoriasis.

**Shadow and Growth Points**

Impatience
Anger and violence
Arrogance
Addiction

## Regenerator (Kapha) Vikriti

Due to their elemental composition (earth and water), Regenerators tend to easily stagnate and develop sluggishness, congestion, heaviness, and lethargy in body and mind. They are prone to all diseases of excess: obesity, diabetes, high cholesterol, fibroids, cysts, or tumors. If they overconsume sugar and refined carbohydrates, Regenerators can be prone to (fungal) infections and candida.

### *Digestion and Metabolism: Sluggish and Slow*

Regenerators have a passion for food and tend to overindulge way beyond their actual digestive capacity and modest metabolic needs. While they can easily skip meals and feel great when fasting or cleansing, they often resist doing so because of their deep emotional connection to food. Regenerators eat for pleasure and comfort, not hunger. They are emotional eaters, tending toward binge eating sweets and junk foods, especially when upset, stressed, or depressed. This leads to sluggishness, stagnation, excess weight, obesity, and diabetes.

### *Energy, Stamina, and Sleep: Lazy and Lethargic*

Out of all constitutions, Regenerators have the greatest stamina and endurance, which, if underutilized, leads to low energy, heaviness, sluggishness, laziness, and depression. A Regenerator loves sleeping (almost as much as eating), but their body thrives on less sleep. In general, they can feel dull and sluggish in the mornings, especially when sleeping in too late. They do much better waking up before sunrise, when the atmosphere is lighter and clearer (Vata time) and supports alertness and freshness.

### *Mental-Emotional: Stuck and Paralyzed*

Psychologically, when out of balance, Regenerators' biggest challenge is feeling stuck, stagnant, and depressed. They do not like to change and can be quite stubborn and set in their ways. Emotionally sensitive and easily hurt, when they're out of balance, they easily slip into depression, feeling paralyzed, or wallowing in self-pity.

### *Relationships: Clingy and Needy*

Out of balance or when pushed and challenged, the cheerful, easygoing, and calm Regenerator can become stubborn, gloomy, and passive-aggressive. Emotional and sensitive as they are, Regenerators can be hurt easily and hold grudges over a long time. If they feel insecure, Regenerators can also become clingy, needy, and possessive. Codependency is a shadow of Regenerators, and they do well finding their internal strength and independence.

### *Disease Pattern: Stagnation and Congestion*

Regenerators' disease pattern is based on excess (overeating, oversleeping, underexercising), which leads to stagnation and congestion. Diseases and imbalances such as high cholesterol, heart disease, diabetes, edema, fibroids, and benign tumors are all related to excess.

#### Shadow and Growth Points

Attachment
Greed
Stubbornness
Codependency

## Coming Back to Balance

Remember that your vikriti is not a fixed diagnosis but a reflection of your current state—a dynamic expression of how life, environment, habits, and emotions shape your inner landscape. The beauty of Ayurveda lies in its understanding that imbalance is not failure; it's feedback. It shows us where we've drifted from our natural rhythm and offers a map back to balance. With awareness and small, consistent choices—food, rest, boundaries, breath—we can shift our trajectory. Instead of trying to "correct" ourselves, we learn to realign. We evolve not by becoming someone else but by becoming more deeply ourselves, day by day.

# Part Two

## Ancient Longevity Secrets for Modern Times

### Harness Your Body's Inbuilt Ability to Flow, Transform, and Regenerate

All of life is choreographed beautifully by the macro movements of flow (kinetic energy), transformation (thermal energy), and regeneration (potential energy). In nature, these forces are embodied in the sun, moon, and wind. In Vedic mythology, they are represented by Surya, the god of the sun, as a symbol of vitality, strength, and enlightenment; Chandra, the god of the moon, known for his gentle and soothing nature; and Vayu, the god of the wind, believed to control the movement of air, life force (prana), and the seasons. When those three forces (or gods) work together harmoniously, our universe—and with it, life—is sustained.

#### *If We Are Plugged In, We Thrive*

We humans are deeply connected to these cosmic cycles. It is the energetic forces of the doshas—Vata as flow or movement, Pitta as transformation, Kapha as regeneration—that directly plugs us into the universe. Just like life is sustained by the cycles of the sun, moon, and wind, so do the doshas enable our bodies to maintain a stable internal environment. From a Western physiological point of view, this means that your body is constantly adjusting its pH, electrolytes, temperature, blood pressure, heart rate, and many other variables to maintain a state of equilibrium, despite changes in the external environment (homeostasis). This ensures that your body fluids are not freezing even though it's -15°C outside. Ayurveda extends this principle of homeostasis to the doshas and their buffering effect on the body.

### *The Secret Key to Excellence and Wellness*

With this in mind, we will dive right into the ancient masters' key to health, excellence, and longevity. Whether we barely make it through the day or live a life full of energy, focus, and meaning; develop chronic disease or radiate well-being; age prematurely or gracefully with vitality and wisdom is largely determined by three crucial factors: our ability to flow, transform, and regenerate. In the upcoming chapters I will show you how to master these three processes. First, the Ayurvedic daily and seasonal routines and practices enable you to synchronize with the (circadian) rhythms of nature, and by doing so, you optimize flow instead of swimming upstream. Second, you ignite your internal digestive, metabolic, and intellectual power, which guarantees that everything you take in (food, thoughts, emotions) is properly digested and transformed. Lastly, you make sure that Flow and Transformation are buffered by your internal fluids (*rasa*, or lymph), which, like a clear mountain stream, will nourish and regenerate all the vital processes, cells, and organs, as well as your nervous system.

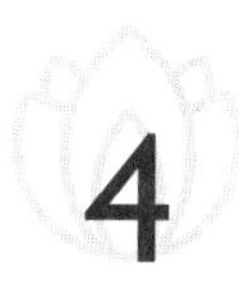

# Hack 1: Flow

Reset Your Circadian Rhythm

## Why Syncing Yourself with Nature Is Crucial: An Ayurvedic and Western Medicine Perspective

### *The Better We Flow, the Healthier We Are*

Nature is all about Flow. Energy flows continuously and incessantly in a cyclical—rather than linear—manner, where each cycle is a microcosm of the next. Just think about the rotation of the earth on its axis causing the circadian cycle of day and night. Rhythmically, sunlight and activity (yang) give way to the darkness of night, where the energy of sleep, stillness, and regeneration (yin) prevails. Embedded in the day and night cycles is also the ebb and flow of the doshas, energetic principles of movement, transformation, and rebuilding. While modern science, most notably research on the circadian rhythm, is only now beginning to understand exactly how important it is for the body to stay in sync with nature, Ayurveda has touted the importance of a connection with nature's cycles for millennia because its scientific model is based on the intrinsic link between macrocosm (our environment) and microcosm (the body).

### *Do as Nature Does: When the Sun Is Up, Don't Sleep; When the Sun Is Down, Don't Eat*

Attunement of our bodies to the external environment is essential for balance, vitality, and health. Just like animals come out in the early morning and go to sleep as the sun sets, you too are deeply connected to the day-and-night cycle. In fact, there is a beautiful saying I heard recently in India: *When the sun is up, don't sleep; when the sun is down, don't eat.* If you just follow this one simple bit of advice, you've already become a superb biohacker. And the emerging science of circadian medicine strongly supports this ancient wisdom. Your body is naturally affected by the light around you. We are diurnal beings. When the sun is up, your energy peaks and your melatonin levels decrease. As the sun goes down, your energy depletes and your melatonin levels rise to prepare you for sleep. Unfortunately, today we see an increasing incidence of genes having literally lost their ability to attune to the natural circadian cycles of nature. Many people—especially those of us living in big cities, working in offices with artificial light, or working at home in front of computer screens—are now diagnosed with what some physicians are calling a "nature-deficit disorder."

### *Plug Into the Seasons*

Along with the cycles of the doshas and day and night, we are subject to the seasonal cycle. The dormant energy of winter bursts forth in spring with new growth, it matures and peaks in summer, then it yields to the harvest of autumn, only to again surrender to the darkness and stillness of winter. Each season brings with it different energetic qualities, which we can harness and cultivate to optimize and recalibrate our own internal climate.

### *The Wisdom of Life Stages*

Along with day and night and the seasons, we have the cycle of life—from birth to childhood, teenage years to middle age, old age to death, and—possibly—back to rebirth. Each segment of our life holds an energetic quality. Childhood is all about growth, which is anabolic and builds Kapha or Regenerator energy. Adulthood is all about achieving and transforming (building a family and/or a career), which is the driven Pitta or Transformer energy. Old age is all about gradual decline—letting go and preparing to die while crystallizing our youthful juiciness into wisdom and compassion—which is dominated and orchestrated by the light and subtle Vata or Mover energy.

### *Ancient Technologies*

*Dinacharya*, *ratricharya*, and *ritucharya*—the Ayurvedic practices of morning, nightly, and seasonal routines—are powerful ancient tools designed to reconnect us to these natural cycles that are wired into our DNA but we have lost connection to. These practices recalibrate us and plug us back into the hardwired genetic coding for health and well-being. I am deliberately devoting quite some time and space in this book to explain to you the beautiful logic and wisdom behind these ancient technologies. For now, just *flow* with me. In this part of the book, I will guide you step by step in how to incorporate these practices into your daily life.

## How to Flow: Detox Daily with Ayurvedic Morning Routines (*Dinacharya*)

Highly successful people often credit their accomplishments to a morning practice. Why? Because the way you start your day determines how the rest of the day flows. You may think you don't have the time, but I can tell you from two decades of clinical and personal experience, with a morning routine you make *more* time for the rest of your day because you are more grounded, focused, and effective. You are in the flow instead of rowing upstream.

### *Turn On Your Brain*

Dinacharya polishes our senses and sense organs. While we rarely think about our senses—eyes (seeing), ears (hearing), nose (smelling), tongue (tasting), and skin (touching)—until they start failing us when we age, the yogis long ago realized that control over and sharpening of the sense organs is fundamental to mental mastery. That is why, in Sanskrit, the sense organs are called wisdom instruments: *jñana-indriyas (jñana*, "wisdom"; *indriya*, "faculty" or "instrument"). Our senses are how we interact with the world, how we make "sense" of it. Senses are what interface between the outside world and our inner world of mind and soul. Sharp senses equal a sharp mind.

## Eight Simple Hacks to Get Into Flow

Below is a little preview of the dinacharya hacks for you. Please don't panic. You will see that you can pick and choose, adding these routines slowly one by one.

1. Rise and Shine
2. Oral "Car" Wash
3. Hydrate
4. Perfect Poop
5. Scrub and Lube
6. Sinus Tune-up
7. Move, Breathe, and Flow
8. *Brrrhhhh* . . . Contrast Shower

## Rise and Shine

If there were a magic pill that would allow everyone to uplevel their creative powers, enhance metabolic activity, lower stress, reset their body's natural sleep-wake cycle, and help them feel more energized and vital throughout the day, the pharma industry would be all over it. You don't even need a pill. Just one simple circadian shift toward waking up early can change your entire biochemistry. Let me explain.

### *Harness the Time of Brahma Muhurta*

According to ancient texts, the secret to health and longevity is waking up *before* the sun rises, during what is called *Brahma muhurta*, or "the time of Brahma (or Creator)." Brahma muhurta is a time of day that is considered highly auspicious in many Vedic traditions—no wonder it is called the time of the Creator. This is the period starting ninety-six minutes before sunrise, when dark turns into light and a new day is on the cusp of being born.

> The healthy person should get up (from bed) during Brahma muhurta, to protect his life.
>
> —*Ashtanga Hridayam, Sutrasthana* 2.1A

According to Vedic belief, the veil between the mundane and subtle worlds lifts during this time. In the silence of early morning, when the air is fresh and the mind is still and calm, you are more likely to access your connection to the depth and mystery of life beyond groceries and to-do lists. By waking up during this time, you can take advantage of these natural qualities of clarity and stillness to gain a physical, mental, and spiritual buffer—and you are much less likely to rush through the rest of your day scattered and unfocused.

While not all of us will make it out of bed in summer by 4 a.m., just remember that a morning routine is established ideally during Vata time, just before sunrise. This helps to remove stagnation, ground the volatile Vata energy, and allow our energy to flow smoothly and freely. When our energy is balanced, our mind becomes centered, and we are more productive, focused, and resilient to stressors.

While sunrise varies according to the seasons, as a general guideline, Mover types should get up before 7 a.m.; Transformers, before 6:30 a.m.; and Regenerators, before 6 a.m. In winter, with sunrise delayed, we also tend to rise a little later. My teacher, Dr. Vasant Lad, used to teach that cholesterol levels and platelet counts stay low—thus preventing high cholesterol and heart disease—when waking up early, before sunrise, when the heavy Kapha energy sets in.

### *Early Sunrays Are Golden Nectar*

In fact, according to ancient Vedic texts, early morning sunrays on your eyes and skin are not only a major source of optimal mood and vitality but can cure a whole range of diseases. Today even, many vaidyas (Ayurvedic physicians) will advise cancer patients to sit in the early morning sun, absorbing its vital rays. Early-morning sun exposure and its resulting increased melatonin production is now increasingly investigated by Western scientists and oncologists for prevention and treatment of cancer.[1]

### *Ancient Wisdom Backed Up by Neuroscience*

Furthermore, the booming field of neuroscience shows that the amount of early (!) daylight exposure you get is crucial in maintaining a normal circadian rhythm.[2] The neuroscience rock star Andrew Huberman advocates going outside and viewing sunlight, without sunglasses, within an hour of waking up (preferably within five to ten minutes of awakening). This primes you to get ready for the day by triggering the release of dopamine and cortisol, which promote wakefulness and the ability to focus throughout the day. It also stimulates the release of serotonin, your feel-good neurotransmitter that regulates mood, appetite, and memory. Serotonin is also a precursor to melatonin, known as your "sleep hormone." When you are exposed to sunlight in the morning, shortly after waking up, your nocturnal melatonin production occurs sooner, and you can enter into sleep more easily at night. Melatonin has a range of effects on the brain, from improving sleep to synchronizing your biological clocks and lowering stress reactivity. Lastly, early-morning sun exposure stimulates the skin to produce vitamin D, which by itself modulates hormones and enzymes that affect almost all organ systems of the body, including the heart, blood, bones, immunity, and neuromuscular health.

## Oral "Car" Wash

### *Tongue Scraping: Why You Need to Remove Your Tongue Coating in the Morning*

Scraping your tongue (*jihva nirlekhana*) in the morning is just as essential as brushing your teeth. Overnight, the body detoxifies. As a result, bacteria and toxins (*ama*) build up on the surface of your tongue, visible in the morning as a whitish and thick tongue coating. This is one of the reasons you get (bad) morning breath. If you do not scrape off these toxins, your tongue absorbs them and they reenter your gastrointestinal tract and general circulation.

But instead of wildly scrubbing the tongue with your toothbrush, which does not clean the surface efficiently and often can injure the delicate taste buds on the surface, you can use a tongue scraper (or a spoon) to scrape your tongue from the back forward, until you have scraped the whole surface three to four times. This practice improves your oral health and prevents gum infections and recessions.[3] It also stimulates and kick-starts your internal organs, which all have reflexology points on the tongue, thus helping digestion and elimination. Last but not least, it uplevels your taste buds, which are not only present in your oral cavity to detect taste but have also been found in the upper esophagus and stomach, as well as other parts of the digestive system such as the pancreas and liver, where they sense the presence of nutrients and other substances in food and send signals to the brain and other digestive organs to prepare for the incoming food.

Which tongue scraper is best? A stainless-steel tongue scraper is much better than the ubiquitous plastic ones. Copper is balancing for Movers and Regenerators, while stainless steel is balancing for all three constitutions, particularly Transformers.

### *Oil Pulling: Not as Ancient as You May Think*

Oil pulling is an oral care practice usually done first thing in the morning on an empty stomach, by swishing one tablespoon of coconut, sesame, or olive oil in the mouth for ten to twenty minutes, then spitting it out. It is said to improve oral health by decreasing bacterial buildup and superbly strengthening gums and teeth.

**How to Do It.** Oil pulling at first might seem a little strange, but it is quite simple. Here is how to do it:

1. After brushing your teeth and scraping your tongue, place one to two teaspoons of an oil of your choice in your mouth and swish it around, also pulling it through your teeth. You can start with just five minutes, and over time work your way up to twenty minutes.
2. Do not swallow the oil since it is full of toxins and bacteria from the teeth and gums. Also, do not spit it in the sink because over time it will surely clog your drains. After you are done, just spit the oil into a tissue or directly into the trash.
3. Rinse your mouth with warm water.

*Tip:* It is not necessary to sit still while doing oil pulling. I usually do it while walking around or doing my other morning routines such as oil massage, dry-brushing, or shower hydrotherapy.

*Trick:* If oil pulling is difficult for you, you can instead place a few drops of sesame oil on your index finger and rub or massage it gently into your gums for one to two minutes. This is a wonderful alternative way to strengthen gums and teeth.

**Which Oil Is Best?** While sesame oil is traditionally used, many people (me included) find it difficult because it is a thick oil. Coconut oil, which is a lot thinner and has a pleasant taste and additional antibacterial and antifungal properties, is my oil of choice. In Turkey, where olive oil is abundant and native, many people prefer using olive oil.

*Note:* You can upgrade your base oil with one to two drops of essential oil—such as peppermint, lemon, clove, or tea tree—for added antibacterial and anti-inflammatory support.

**Ancient Tradition or New Invention?** While you may have read that oil pulling is an old Ayurvedic tradition, surprisingly it is a recent invention. Nowhere in the classical texts do we find a description of oil pulling as it is practiced today. Instead, the current practice leads back to the Ukrainian Dr. F. Karach, who is said to have introduced oil pulling in 1992. While he claimed that it could cure a variety of illnesses including heart disease, digestive troubles, and hormonal disorders, there are no scientific studies available that support his claim. Nevertheless, he is said to have used the method in his medical practice with great success.

When we look at the Ayurvedic classical texts, we only find references to *gandusa*, which is the practice of holding oil in the mouth without moving it around, while sitting in the sun and after having the neck and shoulders massaged. The oil is held in the mouth until mucous accumulates as well as secretions come out from both nose and eyes. Here is what the classical texts say about *gandusa*:

> Keeping of oil gargle provides strength in jaws and voice, development of face, maximum taste and relish in food. The person practicing this does not suffer from dryness of throat, there is no fear of lip-cracking, teeth are not affected with caries, rather they become firm-rooted. They (teeth) are not painful, nor are they oversensitive on sour-taking, they become able to chew even the hardest food items.
>
> —*Charaka Samhita, Sutrasthana* 5.78–80

Gandusa is practiced with various substances such as oils, ghee, milk, honey water, or even meat juice and animal urine (not for the fainthearted), but most of these are used for specific therapeutic purposes. Of the daily use options recommended, oil is perhaps the most appropriate choice. Whereas gandusa involves holding liquids in the mouth without movement, *kavala*—the other classical practice involving oil in the mouth—involves gargling with the oil or other liquids. Gargling is not part of the current practice of oil pulling. In the classical texts, kavala is advised for diseases of the neck, head, ears, mouth, and throat.

> Gargling with oil removes bad taste, bad smells, inflammation, and feelings of numbness in the mouth and is pleasant, strengthens the teeth, and promotes the natural affinity for food.
>
> —*Sushruta Samhita, Chikitsasthana* 24.8

Today's practice of oil pulling is a hybrid of both gandusa and kavala. And while I doubt it is the panacea for all chronic disease, certainly twenty minutes of daily oil pulling is in my opinion a helpful practice that strengthens gums and teeth, improves oral health in general, lubricates the throat, and can reduce general inflammation in the body.

I find the practice of oil pulling also immensely helpful for people with temporal mandibular junction (TMJ) disorder, who clench or grind their teeth at night. In this condition, people can suffer pain in the jaw and surrounding muscles, discomfort when opening or closing the mouth, a clicking sound when the jaw moves, headaches, or even neck and shoulder pain. Because oil pulling exercises oral muscles and increases blood flow to the area, it can help open stagnation and tightness in the mandibular joint.

## Hydrate

During sleep overnight, your body becomes dehydrated. So instead of starting the day with coffee or tea, which drains kidney energy and stresses the adrenals, make it a habit to start your day with warm water. Ayurveda recommends starting your day with a hot drink because it is more hydrating and cleansing than cold beverages—think about the difference between washing your dishes with cold versus hot water. Ayurveda is a big fan of sipping on hot water even throughout the day because it flushes your lymphatic system, removes endotoxins (*ama*), stimulates digestion, kick-starts metabolism, and hydrates deep tissues.

### *Lemon-Honey Water Cleanses Liver and Intestines*

You can even add a squeeze of lemon (and, if you are not intermittent fasting, honey) to a cup of warm water for increased liver and bowel support, and to help eliminate excess Kapha or mucous in the morning. If you add honey, remember to keep your water below 40°C because heat destroys honey's vital enzymes and, according to Ayurveda, makes it toxic.

### *Upgrade: Copper Water*

You may have heard of the Ayurvedic practice of storing water in a copper cup overnight and drinking that copper water first thing in the morning. In addition to copper's proven antibacterial effect, copper water is said to have many other health benefits, including digestive and metabolic support, improved immunity, and better skin and thyroid health. While it certainly needs further scientific investigation, we know that copper is an essential nutrient necessary for maintenance of many body systems, including the immune and digestive systems. I don't advise following the current fashion of carrying around copper water bottles and continuously drinking from that bottle due to the danger of excess copper buildup. Instead, you can drink about one cup in the morning safely and effectively.

## Perfect Poop

It makes sense that before you put any new gas—that is, food—in your tank, you make sure it is emptied first. While you should have a natural bowel movement in the morning, nowadays many people are clogged up and constipated. Ayurveda is obsessed with your bowel movements (BM) because when and how you eliminate; the consistency, color, and smell of the stool; and whether it floats or sinks (yes!) gives us a lot of insight into your digestive power and the health of your microbiome. Remember, if you are not pooping effectively, you become backed up, and wastes and toxins start to accumulate. Over time, this will affect other organs, such as your liver or brain. Recent research on Parkinson's disease, for example, suggests that constipation may be an important preceding factor in the development of the disease.[4]

A healthy BM is easy to pass, well-formed or smooth (like a ripe banana), has a light brown color, no offensive odor, does not stick to the toilet, and floats. Don't be embarrassed if you're not there yet. That's your starting point.

### Top Five Poop Hacks

1. **Go simple.** Eat simple, easy-to-digest foods that are tailored to your constitution, imbalance, and/or season.
2. **Hydrate.** Drink plenty of (warm) water throughout the day to support hydration and elimination.
3. **Move.** Engage in regular exercise or physical activity to help tone muscles, increase circulation, and promote healthy elimination.
4. **Chill.** Reduce stress, which can tighten muscles and negatively impact digestive function.
5. **Bulk up.** Use natural plant fibers such as psyllium, chia, or flaxseeds, and plenty of fiber-rich fruits, vegetables, and whole grains to facilitate bowel motion.

### *Try Triphala*

Triphala is probably Ayurveda's most famous herbal formula. It is a superb bowel cleanser that also promotes cellular rejuvenation and longevity. Literally meaning "three fruits" (*tri*, "three"; *phala*, "fruits"), Triphala is a traditional Ayurvedic blend consisting of three dried and pulverized fruits: amalaki (*Emblica officinalis*), bibhitaki (*Terminalia bellirica*), and haritaki (*Terminalia chebula*). Each fruit balances one of the doshas, making it an excellent choice for almost everyone. My teacher, Dr. Vasant Lad, used to say that Triphala is like your mother; she should always be by your side. While I may not agree with the mother part, Triphala is indeed one of the few herbal supplements that can be taken by old and young continuously throughout life.

Triphala's claim to fame is as a laxative and gentle bowel tonic because it also supports absorption and assimilation of nutrients and promotes a healthy gut flora. But its potency and effect go way beyond your digestive tract. As a powerful antioxidant and anti-inflammatory, it detoxifies and rejuvenates tissues all the way down to the cellular level.

## Scrub and Lube

Did you know that your skin is the largest organ of the human body, covers an average of 15 to 20 square feet, and weighs roughly 5.5 pounds? Your skin is not just one unified layer but consists of three main layers: the epidermis (outermost layer), which provides a protective barrier against the environment; the dermis (mid-layer), which contains connective tissue, blood vessels, and sweat glands; and the subcutaneous tissue, the deepest layer that consists of fat and connective tissue. Together, these layers perform a multitude of functions such as protecting the body against the environment and regulating body temperature and sense perception. The skin even has its own microbiome and immune system that promotes skin health, fights off infections, and maintains a healthy barrier.

### *Scrub*

Dry-brushing is a modern or updated version of the ancient Ayurvedic technique *udvartana*, a dry-powder massage where a mix of powdered herbs or pulses is rubbed all over the body. Often prescribed in Regenerator disorders such as obesity, cellulite, or lymphatic stagnation, udvartana is excellent for exfoliating dead skin cells, increasing circulation, strengthening joints and muscles, and boosting lymphatic flow and drainage. Since it is a messy affair and best experienced with the help of a therapist, I prefer the simple, updated technique of dry-brushing, which is easy and foolproof.

#### WHY SHOULD YOU DRY-BRUSH?

- **Exfoliates:** Dry-brushing removes dead skin cells, which brightens and smooths out your skin.
- **Stimulates lymphatic flow:** Dry-brushing helps stimulate the lymphatic system, promoting detoxification and reducing the risk of lymphatic stagnation.
- **Improves circulation:** Dry-brushing helps to improve circulation, which can increase blood flow to the skin and improve skin nutrition and health.
- **Ignites metabolism:** Dry-brushing stimulates the metabolic fire in your adipose tissue (*meda dhatu agni*) to work more efficiently, thus helping to reduce fat as well as counter cellulite.

**Which Brush Should You Use?** To start dry-brushing, you just need a natural-bristle brush and five to ten minutes of time. Your brush should be on the soft side; it should never leave red marks or scratches. For people with certain skin conditions such as eczema, psoriasis, and rosacea, as well as in Mover types with extremely dry skin, dry-brushing is better replaced with *abhyanga*, or gentle oil massage.

**How to Do It—Don't Scrub Randomly.** When you start dry-brushing, it is important to understand that the lymphatic system flows in a particular way. It is vital to brush in the direction of lymphatic flow, toward the lymph nodes, to effectively increase flow and avoid stagnation.

1. Start brushing on your lower abdomen. First, below your belly button, brush in small strokes down toward your groin on the left and right with five to ten strokes. Then move above your belly button and brush up toward your heart and armpits with about five to ten strokes.
2. Next, brush the upper quadrant of your torso from the sternum outward with small strokes toward the closer armpit.
3. Now brush the upper arm in small strokes toward your armpit. Then do the same on the lower arm and then hands. Then work your way back up the arm, again with small strokes toward the armpit, starting with your hands, lower arm, then upper arm. Repeat the same on the other side.
4. For your legs, start with the upper leg and brush in small strokes toward the groin. Remember to work all around your leg. Then do the same with your knee, lower leg, ankle, and foot. Then work your way back up the leg starting with your foot and ankle, then lower leg, knee, and upper thigh. Remember to get around your entire leg and continue to brush toward your groin. Repeat on your other leg.

### *Lube Up*

Oil is widely respected in Ayurveda. Unlike its long-standing reputation as evil in the West, Ayurveda holds that oil, when prepared and used properly, is an unrivaled medicinal substance. The Sanskrit word for "oil," *sneha*, also means "love" (literally it means "to hold together or bind"). So, this Sanskrit term describes the smooth, binding, and unifying properties of fats and oils, which makes them so nourishing and medicinal.

> Just as a pitcher, the dry skin of the body, and an axis of a cart become strong and resistant through the regular application of oil, so by the massage of oil the whole human body becomes strong and the skin smooth. It becomes nonsusceptible to diseases of vata and resistant to exhaustion and exertion.
>
> —*Charaka Samhita, Sutrasthana* 5.85–86

**Eight Reasons to Oil Up Daily.** While it may at first sound strange to you, according to the ancients, there are innumerous benefits of daily applying oil to the body (*abhyanga*). Oiling up

1. Lubricates skin and prevents wrinkles and sagging
2. Imparts softness, flexibility, strength, and glow
3. Gives tone and vigor to the *dhatus* (tissues)
4. Increases circulation and supports detoxification
5. Increases longevity and prevents aging
6. Strengthens the body's tolerance and immunity
7. Nourishes and calms the nervous system
8. Benefits sleep (especially when practiced at night)

**How to Do It.** You can choose to do your abhyanga right after dry-brushing in the morning. Ideally you take at least fifteen to twenty minutes to make sure the oil can deeply penetrate and nourish all layers of your skin. If you are a Mover type with exceptionally dry skin, you can perform abhyanga after your shower and the skin will just soak up all the oil.

1. Make sure the room where you plan to do your self-massage (most likely your bathroom) is warm. Use an old towel that you do not mind staining with oil and place it on the floor. You can choose to sit or stand on it while you do the massage.
2. Place about one ounce of oil in a squeeze or glass bottle (if you are not using up all the oil, you can warm it again the next day). Put the bottle in a bowl of hot water until the oil is warm.
3. Apply warm oil generously to all parts of your body with gentle strokes. Once applied evenly, you can start massaging the oil into the entire body with a little more pressure.
4. While oil massaging, you always begin at the extremities (hands and feet) and work your way toward your heart. Use long strokes on the limbs, and circular strokes on the joints.
5. Then move to the center of your body and massage your abdomen and chest in clockwise and circular motions. On your belly, follow

the path of the large intestine, moving up the right side (ascending colon), then across (transverse colon), and down on the left (descending colon). Make sure to give a little extra "lube and love" to your head, ears, and feet.

6. While this routine should take you roughly fifteen to twenty minutes, you can do a short tour daily and the long, luxurious version once or twice a week.

**Turbo Version.** If your mornings are already tight and rushed, you can do a mini abhyanga of your head, ears, and feet only. This is an amazing shortcut because, according to the classical texts, the head, ears, and feet have the most important areas with lots of acupressure (*marma*) points and the most nerve endings. If you are short on time in the morning, you can do a full session before bed for a deeper, more restful sleep.

**Upgrade.** Did you know that the potency of sesame oil is enhanced by first *curing* it? Curing sesame oil is an ancient technique that is used to purify the oil and make it more easily absorbable by the skin. During this process, the oil is slowly heated to 100°C and then allowed to cool. Some Ayurvedic brands offer ready-cured oils for purchase, but you can easily cure your own at home. Here is a simple way to do it:

1. Place your sesame oil (ideally organic and cold-pressed) into a pot without a lid and add a few drops of water. Keep the heat on the lowest flame possible to not burn the oil.
2. Once the oil reaches 100°C, the water drops in the oil will begin to sputter. It means your oil is ready.
3. Turn off the heat and allow it to cool completely.
4. Voilà, your oil is "cured." You can pour it back into its original container or any dark glass bottle of your choice.
5. Remember to always store your oils in a dark and cool place and use them up within six months.

## Sinus Tune-Up

Your nose is a direct route to your brain and a doorway to your consciousness. The yogis long ago knew about the deep interconnection between our breathing, prana (our oxygen-carrying life force), our nervous system, and our mental state. They cultivated elaborate techniques of breath manipulation (pranayama) to intentionally affect the body's autonomic nervous system. This way, they were able to boost vital functions such as oxygen supply, lung capacity, heart rate, and immunity, and alter their state of mind. Through breathwork, they improved cognitive function and mental clarity and deepened their meditation practice. My dear teacher, Dr. Vasant Lad, who in his eighties still travels the world teaching students and seeing patients, ascribes his robust health and incredible vitality to a daily pranayama practice.

### *Two Easy Ways to Unblock Your Nose*

Since the boom of the Wim Hof breathing method, as well as James Nestor's groundbreaking book *Breath: The New Science of a Lost Art*, breathwork has gained popularity as a powerful tool for improving physical and mental health. Yet most of my patients have chronically blocked sinuses and a hard time breathing properly even in their daily life. So, if you want to start working with your breath to more effectively uplevel your health, the first step is to make sure your nose is clear and not clogged with "gunk." That is why I find the following two simple Ayurvedic techniques indispensable.

**Nasal Rinse (*Jala Neti*).** Those of you with allergies and chronic sinusitis may already be familiar with a sinus rinse or nasal irrigation (*jala neti*). This technique uses a neti pot, a small teapot-shaped vessel, to wash or rinse the nose with salt water. The flow of salt water through the nasal passage helps to flush out dirt, airborne allergens (dust and pollen), pollutants, and bacteria-filled mucous. This is a lifesaver, especially when you have congestion and a lot of mucous from allergies or a cold.

*Tip:* Neti after airplane trips. While I do not struggle with congestion usually, I still use the neti pot for cleansing after airplane trips and as a preventive measure during flu season, when I have been in contact with lots of people with sniffles. Remember that viruses and bacteria enter our body through the mucous membranes of our mouth and nose, so regular nasal irrigation (as well as gargling with salt water) directly prevents viruses and bacteria from lodging and entering our body.

### How to Do Neti

1. Fill your neti pot with a warm saline water solution: one-half to one teaspoon of sea salt to one cup lukewarm water. Stir well to make sure all the salt dissolves into the water.
2. Over the bathroom sink, tilt your head to one side and let the water run through the nostril that is facing up, which then starts trickling out from the other nostril.
3. Repeat on the other side.

*Tip:* If you have sinusitis with green or yellow mucous, you can also add a quarter teaspoon turmeric to your saline solution as a great antibacterial support.

**Nasal Oleation (*Nasya*).** The practice of *nasya*, my personal favorite, is so important that it made it into what I call the "Great Five," the five fundamental cleansing techniques used in panchakarma (*pancha*, "five"; *karma*, "action"), the famous Ayurvedic detoxification protocol. Nasya involves administering herbal oils, powders, or decoctions through the nostrils. It is used to clean out mucous and toxins that have accumulated in the head and neck region, specifically the nostril and sinuses, as well as the mouth and throat. Many Ayurvedic companies have their own herbal formulations, but in general, oil- or ghee-based products such as *anu thailam* or *brahmi ghee* are considered among the most common and available formulations.

Regular nasya is used to not only clear but also lubricate the delicate membranes of the sinuses, which makes them more resilient against foreign invaders. Additionally, nasya has a long history in Ayurveda of being used to treat a wide range of neurological diseases, including migraines, epilepsy, dementia, Parkinson's disease, or MS. I find it superb for mental clarity and focus in the morning, and as a calming treatment before bed (*shamana nasya*) to promote sound and restful sleep and reduce snoring and sleep apnea.

#### How to Do Nasya

1. Comfortably lie down on your back and tilt your head back so that your nostrils open toward the ceiling.
2. Place two to three drops of nasya or plain sesame oil in your right nostril. Close your left nostril and take a big sniff in through the right.
3. Repeat on the other side, then rest for a few minutes, allowing the nasya to penetrate.

*Tip:* Nasya is best done lying down. If you are outside or on an airplane and lying down is not possible, you can also do it sitting with your head tilted back.

## Move, Breathe, Flow

### *Move*

After elimination, cleansing routines, and hydration, I recommend you take at least fifteen minutes to move and shake your body. Put on your favorite music and groove. What kind of movement you do—dancing, stretching, yoga, walking, or running are all fantastic—is not as important as doing it with joy and consistency. Movement is life, and stagnation is the beginning of disease. Just think of the natural flow of a river. Moving water stays clear, but as soon as it pools and stagnates, it becomes a breeding ground for debris and bacteria.

**Oxygenate Your Cells.** According to Ayurveda, morning is the best time to exercise to counter stagnation that often comes with the heavy Kapha energy that lingers after waking (6 a.m.–10 a.m.). Moreover, your body is naturally stiffer in the morning, after not moving for a long period during sleep, and as a result, the circulation of blood, lymph, and fluids is more stagnant. Remember, movement paired with deliberate and conscious rhythmic breathing is a fantastic way to pump fresh oxygen into your cells and get yourself ready to flow through the rest of your day.

**China's Kung Fu Grandpas.** I remember very vividly from my time spent in Beijing many years ago that on my regular morning walks through Temple of Heaven Park, I was amazed to see crowds of elderly people groove together, practicing an eclectic mix of tai chi, 1980s-style aerobics, and square dancing. Dancing was hugely popular, accompanied by loud music blasting from speakers. It was hilarious and very moving to see these elders collectively having fun and building purpose and connection. One group, the so-called Kung Fu Grandpas/Grannies (which I have only seen on social media), became so famous that their videos went viral on Chinese social media platforms. You can still find a few videos on YouTube of these agile gray panthers displaying incredible flexibility and strength. They're proof that it doesn't matter what age or level of fitness you are, you can find a way to make movement a fun and energizing part of your daily routine. In no time, you will see changes in your level of energy, agility, flexibility, and coordination.

**Caution: More Is Not Necessarily Better.** Keep in mind that whatever form of exercise you choose, more is not necessarily better. While we in the West tend to exaggerate about almost anything we do, including exercise, Ayurvedic wisdom has it that you should always exercise in a way that still allows you to breathe through your nose, and you should stop when sweat forms on your forehead and under your armpits.[5] Otherwise you increase inflammation and stress an often already overburdened adrenal system. This is clearly stated in many of the classical Ayurvedic texts. In *Ashtanga Hrdayam*, *Sutrasthana* 2.14, the ancient Ayurvedic physician Vagbhata said, "Those who indulge daily in too much of physical exercise, keeping awake at nights (loss of sleep), walking long distances, sexual intercourse, too much of laughing, speaking, and such other strenuous activities perish, just as a lion after vanquishing an elephant." Here, a lion is able to vanquish or kill an elephant but soon afterward dies due to severe strain and consequent exhaustion. Similarly, while initially we may feel good from overly strenuous exercise, over time we are harming the body through excessive physical strain.

**What Is the Best Exercise?** Here are some of my favorite ways of moving for the different body types:

Movers, as their name indicates, are pretty good at moving and grooving naturally. They love to be active, and their challenge will be to not push too hard or overstress an already hypernervous and hypermetabolic system. The sweet spot for Movers will be between enjoying the inherent mobile nature of their air element while still paying attention to their limits. Flowing vinyasa yoga can alternate with slower and more restorative yoga sequencing or qi gong; light weight and resistance training can be used for grounding, supporting bones, and building muscle; walking, easy jogging, swimming (in summer), and dancing are good general and easily accessible ways of moving.

Transformers, with their desire for challenge, are usually attracted to competitive and adventure sports. There is nothing wrong with that because, again, Transformers naturally thrive on challenge. But maybe kitesurfing, tennis duels, and ultra-triathlons can be countered with softer activities such as yoga and qi gong; walking, biking, and swimming; and more meditative and flow-state-inducing meditative challenges such as freediving.

Regenerators need to move the most. While they enjoy a slower pace and chilling on the sofa much more than being active, too little activity makes them tired, sluggish, heavy, and lazy. But once they get going, they feel lighter, more energetic, and more vibrant. Constitutionally, Regenerators have great endurance and stamina and thrive on more vigorous forms of yoga such as Ashtanga or vinyasa; heavier weight and resistance training; cardio and HIIT.

### *Breathe*

Even though I breathe deeply and consciously when I stretch, run, or do yoga, I nevertheless also like to build into my morning routine a separate ten-minute breathing (pranayama) session. I find that this enables me to center, get in the zone, and sharpen my focus, clarity, and presence for the day ahead. If nothing else, it certainly makes me more resilient to Istanbul traffic.

**Calibrate with Wim Hof.** If you do not have any breathwork or pranayama experience, it may be best to work with a knowledgeable yoga, meditation, or breathwork instructor. Otherwise I find the Wim Hof method—which is basically a combination of different traditional yogic breath techniques—a superfast way to center and calibrate myself for the day.[6] After those ten minutes, sitting quietly for another ten minutes in meditation almost comes naturally. Remember, your breath carries more than just oxygen. It carries prana (or qi), the vital life force or energy that animates all life forms and is responsible for physical, mental-emotional, and spiritual well-being. When prana or qi is stable and flows freely through the subtle energy channels (*nadis*) in the body, it infuses organs and cells with oxygen, energy, and intelligence. Your mind becomes clear and calm, your cells smarter, and your body more resilient.

## Brrrhhhh . . . Contrast Shower

Growing up in Germany, I would often spend winter evenings with friends in the sauna. After, I'd jump into a cold plunge or roll in the snow. It really invigorated me, and I felt my immune system during flu season was stronger because of this habit. If you don't have a sauna at home, alternating hot and cold showers will do the trick.

### *A Cold Shower Easily Replaces Morning Coffee*

Rather than just taking a warm shower, I invite you to try the contrast-shower hydrotherapy method and see if it doesn't replace your need for morning coffee. The reason is simple: When you take a hot shower, the heat causes the blood vessels in your skin to dilate, increasing blood flow and circulation. When you switch to cold, the sudden drop in temperature causes the blood vessels to constrict, which helps flush out waste and toxins from the lymphatic system. Alternating the temperature of the water between hot and cold stimulates blood flow and improves circulation, which in turn helps to improve lymphatic drainage. This is because the lymphatic system relies on the movement of the muscles and the contraction of the blood vessels to help move lymphatic fluid through the body. As a bonus, cold exposure jolts your system into releasing noradrenaline and endorphins, thus boosting mood and energy.

#### How to Contrast Shower

1. Stand under warm water for a few minutes and relax.
2. Then switch the stream all the way to cold for thirty seconds (beginner) and work your way up to two minutes (advanced).
3. If it is difficult at first, take the shower head in your hand and work on one limb (arms or legs) at a time, working your way toward your heart.
4. Repeat for a total of three rounds—two minutes hot, thirty seconds to two minutes cold—and always finish your last round cold.
5. Voilà—no more need for morning coffee.

**Going Cold Turkey.** During the summer season and with strong Transformer and Regenerator constitutions, you can also directly take a cold shower. If you need to adjust gradually, start with thirty seconds and work your way up to two to three minutes.

### All Seasons in a Day: Sync Your Activities with the Doshic Flow

To harmonize with the cycles of nature, remember that during the day, each segment is ruled by alternating Vata, Pitta, and Kapha energy. During those times, each dosha is (naturally) increased, and this cycle can be used for optimal energy and vitality.

Vata: 2–6 a.m./p.m.
Kapha: 6–10 a.m./p.m.
Pitta: 10–2 a.m./p.m.

**Regenerator or Kapha Time (6 a.m.–10 a.m. and 6 p.m.–10 p.m.).** Regenerator or Kapha time (6 a.m.–10 a.m. and 6 p.m.–10 p.m.) is associated with heaviness, stability, and rebuilding. This is a great time, from an Ayurvedic point of view, to exercise because the body is stronger during a time when the dense earth and water elements are activated. And this is exactly why this is not the best time to eat your heaviest meal of the day (breakfast or dinner). It will make you extra heavy and sleepy.

**Transformer or Pitta Time (10 a.m.–2 p.m. and 10 p.m.–2 a.m.).** Transformer or Pitta time (10 a.m.–2 p.m. and 10 p.m.–2 a.m.) is related to digestion, metabolic and intellectual activity, and cleansing. This time is best for focused work and brain power. It is also ideal to eat the biggest meal of the day between noon and 2 p.m. because our digestive and metabolic power (*agni*) is at its peak. Similarly, it is vital to be in bed (and not at a party) before 10 p.m. to ensure efficient detoxification and clearing of metabolic wastes.

**Mover or Vata Time (2 a.m.–6 a.m. and 2 p.m.–6 p.m.).** Mover or Vata time (2 a.m.–6 a.m. and 2 p.m.–6 p.m.) relates to lightness, flow, and movement. That is why getting up before sunrise will make you feel lighter, uplevel your meditation practice, and support proper elimination. If your general energy and vitality is low, you will feel an afternoon slump around Vata time and you may crave stimulants such as coffee or sugar. Better to not give in to those as they will drain an already weakened Mover adrenal system. A ten-minute power nap or a nourishing and energizing drink such as tulsi tea or ginger–goji berry tea is a wonderful pick-me-up for those afternoon slumps.

| Typical Schedule for Each Dosha | | | |
|---|---|---|---|
| | Mover (Vata) | Transformer (Pitta) | Regenerator (Kapha) |
| Wake Up | 6 a.m.–7a.m. | 5:30 a.m.–6:30 a.m. | 5 a.m.–6 a.m. |
| Breakfast | 8:30 a.m. | 9 a.m.–10 a.m. | Skip |
| Lunch | 12 p.m. | 1 p.m. | Brunch/Lunch 11 a.m.–1 p.m. |
| Dinner | 5:30 p.m. | 6 p.m. | 7 p.m. |
| Sleep | 10 p.m. | 10 p.m. | 10:30 p.m. |

## Nighttime Primers (*Ratricharya*)

In the previous section, we learned about the importance of starting the day right through a set of morning routines (*dinacharya*). In this section I want to show you that your day actually starts the evening before. Why? Because our choices in the evening (*ratricharya*) greatly determine how we feel in the morning. I cannot tell you how many clients of mine have gone from snoozing through their alarms and feeling groggy and foggy in the morning to waking up naturally and starting their day feeling like a million bucks—just with a few simple adjustments to their evening routine.

### *Our Ancestors Did It Right*

Prior to electricity, when people were still mostly farmers, their evenings were largely dictated by the natural light of the sun. They ate their main meal when returning from the fields around late afternoon, relaxed with the family, and went to bed shortly after the sun set. With the advent of electricity, however, it was suddenly possible to work, read, eat, and socialize well into the night. This led to a significant shift in the timing of our evening routines, with many people staying up way past their natural circadian wiring.

The end of the day is for winding down. Remember that early evening hours, 6 p.m. to 10 p.m., is Kapha or Regenerator time. Ayurveda recommends using the natural tendencies of Kapha energy—slowness, heaviness, grounding—to wind down, connect with family, reflect on the day, and prime our nervous systems for sleep. But rather than winding down, many of us work long hours or commute from work and return home late. We eat our biggest meal often after 8 p.m., only then to collapse on the sofa and reward (or self-medicate) with Netflix, Instagram, red wine, and chocolate. While this may feel good in the moment, remember that when we go against the natural rhythm of the universe, our body must work twice as hard. We are swimming upstream. The result: In the morning we feel tired and groggy and have difficulty getting out of bed.

### *Three Crucial Sleep Primers*

Ayurveda holds that with a few simple adjustments to your evening routine (*ratricharya*), you can support body and mind to recuperate from the stressors of the day and properly replenish for the day ahead.

1. Eat dinner early and light.
2. Shift your bedtime closer to 10 p.m.
3. Prime your nervous system for winding down.
    a. Unplug
    b. Feet lube
    c. Relax
    d. Sense polishing
    e. Sleep elixir

### *Eat Dinner Early and Light*

Many of us eat late and heavy dinners out of social habit. Gathering the family around the dinner table or going out and socializing over drinks and dinner has become a norm. There is nothing wrong with socializing or family time. On the contrary, this social time and bonding deeply nourish us; we just need to uncouple it from a heavy late meal and too much alcohol.

**Agni Plummets at Night.** In line with the natural circadian wiring, Ayurveda recommends that we eat dinner in the earlier part of the evening, preferably before sunset, but by 7 p.m. at the latest. The evening meal should be much lighter than the midday meal and easy to digest. Think about this: If the body must spend half of the night digesting food, it cannot focus on clearing metabolic wastes and replenishing the organs. Nor can it properly process the mental and emotional strains of the day. Since agni, your internal fire or digestive capacity, is wired into the rhythm of the sun, it peaks at noon and weakens toward evening. This is why Ayurveda does not recommend eating cold and clogging foods such as dairy (cheese, ice cream, milk, yogurt) at night. Similarly, raw food takes more digestive effort to break down and is—at least in winter—better substituted with a bowl of warm soup in the evening. When you eat a solid meal around noon, your agni has plenty of time to digest, metabolize, and transform your meal into energy and healthy tissues. If you eat your biggest meal (late) in the evening, agni gets overwhelmed and undigested food or endotoxins (*ama*) build up in your gut and channels.

**Skip Dinner, Not Lunch.** It is useful to look at the rather old-fashioned name for the last meal of the day: supper. I like to think of it as a "supp"-lemental meal, not as the main event of the day. The word *supper* comes from the Old English word *sop*, which referred to a piece of bread soaked in liquid. Over time, *sop* came to mean the meal itself, particularly the last meal of the day. It was likely influenced by the Old French word *souper*, which also meant to have an evening meal, mostly a bowl of "soup." Interestingly, the word *dinner* used to refer to the main meal of the day, which was usually eaten around noon. Over time, the meaning of *dinner* shifted to refer to the evening meal, while *supper* continued to be used to describe the last meal of the day. Rather than just shifting its meaning, we also shifted the heavier contents of dinner as a main meal to the evening, while skipping lunch or grabbing a quick salad or sandwich. As a result, by the time dinner comes around, we are hangry (hungry and angry), exhausted, and frazzled.

**"Eat Breakfast Like a Yogi, Lunch Like a *Bhogi*, and Dinner Like a *Rogi*."** "Eat breakfast like a yogi, lunch like a *bhogi*, and dinner like a *rogi*": I love this common Indian proverb because, with humor, it summarizes Ayurveda's nutritional philosophy. Eating breakfast like a yogi means that you eat breakfast wisely, according to your unique needs, which are based on your appetite, digestive capacity, and energy requirements of the day. This might be a hearty meal with eggs, greens, and mushrooms if you are hungry and have been physically active; a small breakfast porridge or granola if you do better with simple foods first thing in the morning; or skipping breakfast altogether if you are a Regenerator type or generally have little appetite in the morning. Remember, *breakfast* means breaking the fast of the night, so it should be a light affair unless you eat your first meal closer to noon. *Bhogi* comes from the Sanskrit word *bhoga*, which means "sensory enjoyment or pleasure." A bhogi is someone who lives only for the pleasures of life. Eating lunch like a bhogi means enjoying a full and satisfying meal that may include a variety of different dishes and also harder-to-digest foods such as animal proteins (meat, eggs, fish). *Rogi* comes from *roga*, which means "disease." Eating dinner like a *rogi*, or patient, means to either skip it (if you are not hungry) or have a dinner that is light and easy to digest. Do you remember the foods you crave when you are sick? They are usually light foods such as soups, broths, or steamed veggies—basically anything that is nourishing while not burdening digestion.

**Freeing Up Your Evening.** When you eat an early and simple dinner, it frees up space for other activities such as resting, relaxing, gardening, listening to music, reading, or going for a leisurely evening walk alone or with friends or family. This lets your nervous system recuperate from the stressors of the day and helps you wind down toward sleep instead of hyperstimulating it with watching television, social media scrolling, or intense mental work.

**Intermittent Fasting (IF): The Ancients Were Doing It All Along.** Lastly, one note about the Ayurvedic view on intermittent fasting (IF). Long before IF became a popular biohack, the ancients were already doing it. The yogis in India have eaten only one meal a day for millennia. My main Ayurveda teacher, Dr. Vasant Lad, skips dinner entirely. At the Ayurvedic center in India where I take my students for training, dinner is around 5 p.m. and very light, maybe just kitchari or lentil soup with chapati. In Ayurveda, the concept of intermittent fasting is known as *upavasa*, a practice that involves abstaining from food or reducing food intake for a specific period. This practice is used therapeutically to help remove toxins from the body, improve digestion, and promote mental clarity. Eating an early light dinner around 5 p.m. or 6 p.m. and then fasting for fourteen to sixteen hours before breaking it with a light meal (break-fast) around 9 a.m. the next morning is a fantastic way to give your digestive system a much-needed and complete rest. It also helps to activate your cells' natural intelligence, their inbuilt fire element (*agni*) that ignites them to burn through toxins, scavenge for oxidative damage, eliminate damaged cells, and destroy pathogens.

**Frequent and Late-Night Eating Leads to Inflammation.** Eating too late or too frequently disrupts this inbuilt ability for regeneration and (epi)genetic optimization. Without a sufficient rest phase, food cannot be digested entirely. Undigested gunk (*ama*) makes its way into and around the cells, where it disrupts cellular function, communication, and oxygenation. Instead of smooth energy production and waste elimination, energy now is funneled into cell repair. This provokes an inflammatory immune response. It is an uphill battle, and at some point, the body succumbs to fatigue, dysbiosis, candida, autoimmune conditions, and chronic degenerative disease.

**Why You May Be Doing IF Wrong.** Many intermittent fasters are morning fasters, meaning their sixteen-hour fasting window is between 8 p.m. and 9 p.m. for their last (and often heaviest) meal and noon or 1 p.m. for their first meal of the day. I prefer the Ayurvedic way of a smaller fasting window of twelve to fifteen hours, based on an early dinner at 6 p.m. or 7 p.m. and breakfast early in the day around 8 a.m. or 9 a.m. (especially if you get up before sunrise, around 6 a.m.). This gives you enough time for your morning routines on an empty stomach but ensures your body gets the fuel and grounding needed for the start of the day. Especially for Movers and Transformers, breakfast instead of coffee on an empty stomach prevents them from going into a stress response during a time when cortisol levels are already naturally high. These, of course, are just general guidelines. You want to tailor your fasting program always on individualized practices, based on your unique constitution, strength, imbalance, and current health needs.[7]

**(Intermittent) Fasting According to Your Metabolic Type.** Movers (Vata): Air-predominant individuals (prone to irregular agni, low weight, and depleted energy reserves) do much better with short, gentle fasts of twelve to fourteen hours that do not cause stress to the body. This could be an early dinner between 6 p.m. and 7 p.m. and then breakfast between 8 a.m. and 9 a.m. Longer twenty-four- to forty-eight-hour fasts are helpful only as a mono diet of soup or kitchari fasting.

Transformers (Pitta): Fire-predominant individuals can fast for longer periods than Movers. An early dinner around 6 p.m. and breakfast between 8 a.m. and 10 a.m. is ideal. Once a month they can also do a twenty-four-hour vegetable juice or water fast to counter their tendency toward acidity and inflammation.

Regenerators (Kapha): Earth-dominant constitutions usually thrive on fasting. They do well with only two meals per day and a longer fasting window of sixteen hours. An early dinner around 6 p.m. and late breakfast or brunch around 11 a.m. helps to balance their heavy nature, sluggish digestion, and foggy mind. Regenerators also do well with a weekly twenty-four-hour water fast.

### *Shift Your Bedtime Closer to 10 p.m.*

Sleep is the most innocent creature there is and a sleepless man the most guilty.

—Franz Kafka, *Letters to Milena*

Sleep, untimely, excessive or scanty, will destroy happiness and life itself like the legendary demoness of the night—kalaratri.

—*Charaka Samhita, Sutrasthana* 21.36–38

Long seen as trivial and a waste of time, sleep (*nidra*) is certainly one of, and maybe the most, fundamental factor for health.[8] According to Ayurveda, next to food (*ahara*) and balanced sexuality (*brahmacharya*), sleep is an essential human drive and vital for most physiological and cognitive functions. During sleep, the body and mind are allowed to cleanse, recalibrate, rest, and rejuvenate. From an Ayurvedic perspective, sleep can happen because in the dark and stillness of the night, *tamas* (inertia) is predominant, and the body, sense organs, and mind become heavy and dull—we get sleepy. In the morning, when dawn and sunrise bring *sattvic* (harmonious and balancing) qualities, the senses become active, bright, and energetic and we wake up.[9]

**Sleep Is More Than a Pause Button.** While from the outside, sleep seems nothing more than a pause button for body and mind, on the inside, a busy night shift is taking place. Metabolic wastes are removed, tissues repaired, organs replenished, protein synthesized, and hormones released. At the same time, in the brain, new neural pathways are formed, memory consolidated, and brain synapse signals rebooted.

**Brain Drain.** Recent research has also revealed that the brain detoxifies at night. The glymphatic system, a network of capillaries that constitutes the brain's waste management system, is more active during sleep. Particularly during deep sleep, the flow of cerebrospinal fluid (CSF) through the glymphatic system increases, flushing out waste products and allowing the brain to clear built-up toxins.[10] For all these beautiful processes to work efficiently, Ayurveda recommends being in bed by 10 p.m., at the latest, the start of Pitta time, where your body's inbuilt metabolic fire supports detoxification, waste removal, and rejuvenation. During this time, according to the organ clock, our main detoxifier, the liver, is the most active.

**Dreams Are More Than Random Firing of Neurons.** Finally, sleep and the dream world have long been fascinating and puzzling aspects of our being and the subjects of various spiritual traditions and scientific disciplines. The ancient yogis and many other Indigenous cultures around the world view dreams as another aspect of reality (or another layer of consciousness), where we can receive guidance, release stress, and work through difficult experiences and unprocessed emotions.

In yogic philosophy, dreams are seen as a manifestation of the subconscious mind (*chitta*), which is the storehouse of memories, experiences, and impressions from our past and present lives. The subconscious mind is also believed to contain *samskaras*, deep-rooted mental impressions or tendencies that influence most of our thoughts, emotions, and behaviors. Yogic practitioners believe that by developing awareness of our dreams, we can gain insights into our subconscious mind and the patterns that influence our waking life. They also believe that through certain yogic practices, such as meditation, yoga nidra, or dream yoga,[11] we can purify our subconscious, release negative samskaras, and change deep-seated patterns.

**What Is Your Sleep Pattern?** Healthy and restful sleep should occur naturally. Unhealthy sleep can be too heavy, often due to toxins (*ama*), intoxication (alcohol), or late-night overeating; or it can be too light and interrupted, often due to stress, mental agitation, worry, anxiety, and restlessness. Let's first look at your constitutional tendencies regarding sleep, and later I will give concrete action steps for correcting imbalances.

**Movers (Vata) and Sleep.** Movers' sleep pattern tends to be irregular and light, and even with little sleep, they wake up energetic and bright. Movers often sleep too little for what their nervous systems need for recuperation, which is at least eight hours. Movers have difficulty falling asleep if they are anxious or their minds are too active, or they wake up during Vata time (2 a.m.–6 a.m.), toss and turn, and are unable to go back to sleep.

**Transformers (Pitta) and Sleep.** Transformers generally sleep well and wake up easily and alert. If under deadline pressure or excited about a project, Transformers can get their second wind after 10 p.m. (Pitta time), feeling super productive and focused during this time, and can stay up way past midnight. This, however, especially when it becomes a habit, compromises the extra-nourishing sleep before midnight, which can leave their bodies more acidic and inflamed, and their minds more irritable the next day.

**Regenerators (Kapha) and Sleep.** Regenerators are heavy sleepers and can sleep soundly anywhere and anytime. They love sleeping, but out of all types, they need the least amount of sleep. Usually five to six hours is sufficient for them. The longer that Regenerators sleep and the later they wake up (especially after sunrise, which is the beginning of heavy and grounding Kapha time), the heavier and duller they feel and the harder it is for them to get going.

**Power Naps for Movers and Transformers.** Daytime sleeping should be avoided, except in the case of night-shifters, after physical exertion, when sick or very weak and depleted; and for children. People with Regenerator constitutions or Kapha imbalances should avoid daytime sleep altogether, since it can cause congestion, indigestion, heaviness, edema, lethargy, and headaches. Movers and Transformers can take short, ten-minute power naps after lunch, especially in the heat of summer, preferably lying on their left side to activate right nostril (solar) breathing, which supports digestion.

### *Prime Your Nervous System for Winding Down*

Sleep is considered so fundamental for health and well-being that Ayurveda proposes a separate list of nighttime rituals that help prime our nervous system to wind down and set the stage for optimal sleep.

**Unplug.** I already briefly discussed how overuse of screens and electronic devices in the evening has been shown to disrupt our circadian rhythm or natural sleep-wake cycle and negatively impact the quality of our sleep. This is because the blue light emitted by these devices can suppress the production of the sleep-inducing hormone melatonin, making it more difficult to fall and stay asleep. In my practice, I see many clients with sleep disorders, often due to hyperstimulated nervous systems that lack the *tamas*, or natural heaviness and grounding, for proper deep relaxation and sleep. I recommend disconnecting from all electronics at least one hour—ideally two hours—before sleep. You can read, relax, listen to music, or start preparations for the day ahead. If you absolutely need to use a screen, wear blue-light-blocking glasses or switch your device to "night mode," which favors the less disruptive red and orange hues.[12]

**Feet Lube.** When I was in India for Ayurvedic treatments a few years ago and suffered from bouts of insomnia, the doctors would send two therapists to my room each night to give me a foot massage with warm sesame oil before bed. It was so simple, took at most five minutes, and worked wonders. While back home I did not always have two therapists at hand, a simple three-to-five-minute self-*padabhyanga* (*pada*, "foot"; *abhyanga*, "massage") became a regular part of my evening routine. Think of it like a mini reflexology treatment, where you stimulate pressure points in your feet that are distally connected to your organs. By touching your feet with warm sesame oil—which is heavy, warming, and nourishing—you start moving overactive nervous energy from your head downward into your feet and grounding it into the tamas or stillness of night.

**Tailor and Upgrade Your Oil.** During summer or if you are a Transformer who tends to run hot at night, I recommend using coconut oil for self-padabhyanga. In the other seasons, if you are cold easily and for Movers in general, use warm sesame oil. You may even add one to two drops of lavender or *jatamansi* (Indian valerian or spikenard) essential oil for additional relaxation.

### How to Do It

1. Warm your oil by putting a small bottle with one ounce of your oil of choice in a bowl of hot water for a few minutes.
2. If you are sitting on the sofa or bed, place a small towel under your feet to prevent oil spilling on sheets or cushions.

3. Rub your feet clean with a washcloth soaked in warm water, then start by massaging a small amount of oil into one foot at a time until both feet are equally coated.
4. Treating one foot at a time, progress to massaging your ankle in circular motion; move to the top of the foot, back and forth from the toes all the way to the ankle. Don't forget to include your toes in the massage, squeezing and massaging each toe individually.
5. Lastly, you can use firmer pressure to massage the sole of the foot, including the heel. Find any spots that feel especially tender and linger there a little longer to help break up stagnation. Then move to the other foot and start the same sequence.
6. You can finish by again rubbing your feet clean with a washcloth soaked in warm water or directly putting on a pair of old socks so you can keep all the benefits of the oil on your feet overnight.

**Relax (Breathing, Meditation, Yoga Nidra).** Yoga and Ayurveda both offer a wide range of simple practices that can help relaxation and sleep priming. Breathing routines such as alternate nostril breathing (*nadi shodhana*), humming bee breath (*brahmari*), and box breathing (*sama vritti*) before bed help calm the mind, draw the attention inward, and balance the light and mobile Vata energy that often prevents us from falling asleep easily.

**The Ancient Technology of Yogic Sleep (Yoga Nidra).** If you don't already have a meditation practice that enables you to calibrate your nervous system toward deeper relaxation, I highly recommend trying an ancient practice called *yoga nidra*. Yoga nidra is a form of guided meditation (usually fifteen to twenty-five minutes long) that is practiced lying down and can be used to promote relaxation, reduce stress, and improve sleep. It is sometimes referred to as "yogic sleep" because it induces a state of relaxation so deep and nourishing that it can be as restful as actual sleep. During a yoga nidra practice, you are encouraged to focus your attention on different parts of your body, your breathing, and sometimes also images. This increased self-awareness helps release mental blocks as well as subtle physical tension that keep you from getting a good night's sleep. Yoga nidra is a wonderful method to relax and to improve sleep depth and quality.[13]

**Sense Polishing: Eyes—the Ancient Practice of *Netra Basti*.** The eyes are our window to the world. They orient us and enable us to take in breathtaking colors and incredible beauty. We rely on them more than any other sense. For most of us with office or computer jobs, instead of taking in incredible beauty, our eyes must bear the onslaught of artificial lighting and computer screens, day in and day out, often for hours on end. Our eyes deserve a little love and support. In Ayurveda, the eyes are part of our nervous tissue (*majja dhatu*), which means we can use them to directly influence our nervous system. In the Ayurvedic treatment called *netra basti*, which literally means "eye bath," a small dam of lentil flour dough is formed around both eyes and filled with melted ghee. While the eyes are completely submerged in ghee, the client is asked to frequently blink and open their eyes so that all the nourishing and healing properties of the ghee can penetrate the tissues of the eyes.

**Do-It-Yourself Version.** While you need a qualified therapist for netra basti, there is a similar technique you can comfortably do yourself at home before bed. You may already be using over-the-counter eye drops to soothe dry, irritated, or tired eyes. I would invite you instead to try one drop of pure organic ghee (clarified butter) in each eye right before bed, which is an amazing cooling, soothing, and nourishing treatment. Don't worry when things start looking a little blurry. This just means that enough ghee is coating your eyeballs and ready to nourish your eyes overnight.

### How to Do It

1. Put a small amount of plain ghee into a glass dropper bottle and keep it ready by your bedside. In winter or if your house is very cold, you may need to hold the bottle in your hands for a few minutes so that the ghee melts and is liquid.
2. When you are ready to sleep, before switching off the light, either

sitting or lying, tilt your head back and drop one drop of ghee into each eye.

3. If this is too scary or proves difficult, try massaging a little ghee around the eyes, up to the edge of the lids, and wait until some of the ghee starts to seep into the eyes.

**Sense Polishing: Lubing the Ears—the Ancient Practice of *Karna Purana*.** People are usually skeptical about *karna purana* (*karna*, "ear": *purana*, "to fill"), or ear oiling, but once they try it, they are hooked. This practice involves pouring lightly warmed sesame oil into the ear and letting it absorb for five to ten minutes. I had a client years ago who suffered from insomnia. While we tried everything from changing his diet and optimizing his evening routine to using strong herbal support including ashwagandha and jatamansi (the Indian equivalent to valerian root), it was only after he added karna purana three times per week that he experienced a significant improvement in his sleep. I love doing this practice, especially after traveling and flying or at the end of a long teaching day. Almost effortlessly does this switch my nervous system mode from "tired and wired" to "rest and restore."

### How to Do It

1. With a towel under your head, lie facing up. Tilt your head to one side and start pouring a small amount (roughly one or two teaspoons) of lightly(!) warmed sesame oil into the outer canal of the ear that is facing up. Make sure to fill the canal all the way to the rim. Then you relax and let it absorb for five to ten minutes.
2. Lightly press a folded tissue paper onto the ear and turn your head to the other side so that the oil drains directly into the tissue paper.
3. Repeat on the other side.
4. Initially there may be a slight sensation of fullness, pressure, or discomfort, but quickly this gives way to deep relaxation.

**Poppy-Seed Milk: An Ancient Sleep Elixir.** For deeper sleep and relaxation, you can use this beautiful, medicated poppy-seed milk that is very tasty and nourishing. It is a popular and effective sleep remedy and a staple in many Indian grandmas' households. Combining nutmeg with poppy seeds is especially effective as both herbs by themselves are powerful sedatives but have different action times. Nutmeg needs a few hours before its maximum sedative effect kicks in, so it is a suitable remedy for people falling asleep easily but waking up in the middle of the night. Poppy seeds, on the contrary, are fast-acting, but the action wears off after a few hours, so they are preferred by some of my clients that have trouble falling asleep. By combining the two, you get the benefits of both worlds and a superb sleep combo. You can find the recipe for Deep-Sleep Tonic in the recipe section.

## Living According to Seasons (*Ritucharya*)

As the earth spins around the sun, our spatial relation to it defines how much sunlight we receive. In this way the seasons and changes in nature are produced. Each season brings with it its own unique energy and character. The better we align ourselves with the rhythm and qualities of each season, the less likely we are to become imbalanced. Just as the seasons and their dominant elements change throughout the year, so do our bodies. In fall and early winter (October–January), Vata energy is dominant, and with it, the dry, cold, and light qualities. In late winter and spring (February–May), Kapha is dominant, and with it, the cool, heavy, and moist qualities. In summer (June–September), Pitta energy is dominant, and with it, the hot, light, and sharp qualities. We need to adapt our diet and lifestyle to each season to promote optimal health and avoid imbalance.

### *The Earth Knows Best*

When we look at nature, we see that each season brings us the harvest that balances our body in that season. For example, in fall and winter (Vata season) we find heavier foods such as root vegetables and sturdy winter greens, and a greater emphasis on beans, lentils, nuts, and meat dishes and stews. In spring (Kapha season) we see artichokes, tender greens such as nettles, tart berries, and bitter roots, which are all great liver and gallbladder detoxifiers. In summer (Pitta season), nature provides an abundance of juicy summer fruits, cooling cucumbers, and plenty of fresh aromatic herbs and salad greens.

### *The Problem with Mangoes from Mexico and Strawberries in Winter*

Since most of us no longer exclusively live off the land through farming, we have forgotten how to eat seasonally. Our supermarkets are stocked with the same produce all year round. We now have strawberries, tomatoes, and cucumbers even in the winter season, grown in greenhouses; and tropical fruits such as mangoes and pineapples, not even part of our climate zone but imported from faraway places such as Hawaii or Mexico. In addition, we live in temperature-controlled environments—with heated homes in winter and air-conditioning in the summer—very much removed from the actual temperature and conditions outside. Compare that to a farmer just 150 years ago. Their life was intrinsically woven into the weather pattern and season all year round.

### *How to Realign with the Seasons*

In the following chapter I will show you how to plug into the elements, qualities, and potential of each season so that you can better realign yourself with the cycles of nature. You may already actually be doing some of it intuitively. As the sun returns in the spring after the long, dark winter months, we tune in to the energy of new beginnings and growth. In the summer, we naturally tap into the energy of abundance, passion, and joy. In the fall, we embrace the energy of change, letting go, and transformation. In the winter, we tune in to the energy of rest and introspection.

## Fall and Early Winter: Recalibrate Your Vata

According to the elemental cycles in Ayurveda, fall welcomes the ether and air elements and with them the cold, dry, rough, and light qualities of Vata dosha. Trees start dropping their leaves, days get shorter and nights cooler, scarves replace sunglasses, and warming teas take the place of summer ice-cream fun. We say goodbye to seemingly endless summer days and balmy summer nights, and settle back into school, work routine, and structure.

The transition from summer to fall is a difficult one for me, both physically and emotionally. I long for morning swims in the clear-blue sea, coming back sun-kissed from the beach in the late afternoon, and enjoying warm evenings under the stars. My body struggles to adjust to the cold, dryness starts to creep in, and in my heart a sweet melancholy settles when witnessing nature dying. During this time, more than ever, I look to the ancient Eastern wisdom of the elements—the teachings and practices of Ayurveda and Chinese medicine—to find guidance and support for my body, mind, and spirit through the transformational opportunity that comes with the seasonal change.

### *Do as Nature Does: Prepare for Hibernation*

When we observe nature, the fall season has a clear theme. Just as trees shed their leaves, letting go of what is no longer needed and drawing their essence deep into the roots to hibernate and gather energy in the stillness of winter, we are invited to move inward, slow down, and let go of what may not serve us anymore, whether that is a piece of clothing, a habit, or a relationship. According to Chinese cosmology, fall is ruled by the metal element, which governs the lungs and large intestine. Both are about letting go of what no longer serves ($CO_2$ and feces) so that we can again take in what is nourishing and needed (oxygen and food). If we resist the flow of autumn, we can develop signs of Vata aggravation or metal imbalance, with symptoms such as constipation, asthma, weakened immunity, and susceptibility to colds, cough, and bronchial or sinus infections. There is a saying in Chinese medicine that "wind is the cause of a thousand diseases," which directly corresponds to Ayurveda's teaching that Vata is at the root of almost all diseases. Wind more than any other element can move, enter the body swiftly, and affect organs and channels.

### *Say Goodbye to Smoothies and Salads*

To best adjust to the coldness and dryness that fall brings, it is good to follow a diet that relies more on warm, cooked, and moist or slightly oily foods. As September rolls around, start reducing cold foods, raw salads, and green smoothies, as well as fasting or skipping meals, especially breakfast. Since Vata energy is irregular and mobile, keep regularity (regular meal and bedtimes especially, as well as a set morning routine). From October onward, make sure to stay warm, enjoy regular steam baths, and get plenty of rest. If energy is very low, maybe even nap for ten minutes during Vata time, between 2 p.m. and 4 p.m.

Since the days are getting shorter, start eating your dinner earlier (by 7 p.m. at the latest) and start winding down and going to bed earlier, ideally around 10 p.m. You can drink a cup of warm (almond) milk at bedtime, with poppy seeds and a pinch of nutmeg. This helps calm restless Mover minds and promotes sound sleep.

### *Lube and Ground*

During autumn, you can start supporting your lungs for a healthy winter season by practicing regular breathing exercises such as warming solar breathing (*surya bhedana*) or calming alternate nostril breathing (*nadi shodhana*). A daily meditation practice to calm the mobile Mover mind, even if it is just for ten to fifteen minutes, can make a huge difference. Perform a daily full-body self-massage (abhyanga) with warm sesame oil and a few drops of lavender, rosemary, and ginger essential oils. In addition, if you can schedule a professional massage for yourself once a week, even better. Nothing calms a Mover better than a warm oil massage. Enjoy regular, relaxing, and peaceful walks in nature to calm the mobile body and active mind.

### *Warm Up*

In fall and early winter, wear warming colors such as yellow, orange, red, or black; avoid cooling colors such as gray, white, blue, and green. In your yoga practice, focus on warming flows such as sun salutations (*surya namaskar*) as well as plenty of forward bending and passive inversions such as legs-up-the-wall (*viparita karani*). Be sure to follow activities with sufficient rest. To enhance circulation and digestion, as well as support immunity, drink a warming tea of fresh ginger and goji berries or Chinese red dates.

## Late Winter and Spring: Recalibrate Your Kapha

The winter months, when nature goes into hibernation, are an invitation to tune in to the energetic quality of yin—resting, conserving energy, recharging, and replenishing the resources you have spent throughout the year.

### *Deep Rest Brings New Growth*

The energy of winter is deep and potent. While the earth and trees are barren and seem dead (and it feels like spring and new life will never return), I hold on to the knowing that underneath the surface of rest and stillness, a tremendous amount of work is happening. Only because of the collecting energy and building resources beneath the surface can spring—and with it new growth, rebirth, and fresh starts—happen. In the bigger cycle of life and death, it is only through a continuous cycle of dying and decomposing that new life is nourished and reborn, quite literally.

### *Connect to the Depth of Water*

According to Chinese medicine, winter is ruled by the water element and its related organ, the kidneys. There is depth, darkness, and a great mystery to water. On a recent freediving experience in Bali, as I dived with nothing but my own breath down into the depths of the ocean—first three, then five, then ten, and lastly fourteen meters—I could feel the overwhelming power that comes from the depth of the ocean. Water is one of the most nourishing and essential substances for life, and our bodies are mostly made of it. Over billions of years, we have evolved from water. Just like a barren winter landscape, when you look at the surface of the ocean, not much seems to be going on. But once you dive into it, you discover another world under water brimming with life, the most intense play of colors, incredible grace, and beauty.

### *In Winter We Build and Store*

In Ayurveda, winter is both the time of Vata (early winter) and Kapha (late winter). During this time, we naturally tend to be less active and store heat and fat—and we may also gain a few extra pounds. Due to the external cold, our digestive fire (*agni*) is pushed to the body's core, strengthens and intensifies there, and helps us replenish spent energy, rebuild tissues, and build a fat layer that helps insulate against the cold. As a result, we naturally crave heavier and heartier kinds of foods in wintertime, such as hot soups, bean or meat stews, and root vegetables.

### *How to Avoid Spring Allergies*

Toward the end of winter, however, starting in February and March, the sun regains strength and the weather warms. Just as the snow starts melting in the mountains, similarly the Kapha that has protected us so well in winter—but also led to excess stagnation and mucous—starts to liquify. This can lead to congestion, spring allergies, and spring fatigue, as well as depression. Therefore, it is best to avoid cold and mucous-forming foods (iced drinks, dairy products, sugar, and excess carbohydrates such as bread and pasta). Instead, during this time, support the body's natural cleansing process with a diet that is mostly plant based. Lean toward foods that are light, warm, and stimulating, such as spicy soups and broths; and plenty of fresh greens, nettles, and other liver-cleansing foods, such as artichokes, asparagus, greens, lemons, and radishes. You could even try juice or water fasting for a day or two, which often works wonders in resetting energy and vitality.

### *Why We Often Experience Fatigue and Mood Issues in Spring*

In Chinese medicine, after the darkness and stillness of winter comes spring with the energy of wood and the theme of new growth and rebirth. Think of the energy of a seed planted in spring. All of its effort goes toward rising, pushing through, and orienting itself to the sun for nourishment and growth. Often, however, excess Kapha, stagnation, or mucous blocks and constrains this rising energy. This is referred to as qi stagnation in Chinese medicine, and can manifest emotionally as anger, irritability, mood swings, or depression; and physically as migraines, pain, lethargy, fatigue, and neck and shoulder tension. For women in spring, PMS symptoms can intensify and menstrual cramps worsen.

### *Hit the Gym*

Stimulation and activity in spring is key to beat any lingering stagnation and lethargy, so get up early (ideally before sunrise) and schedule activities and social outings that get you moving instead of lounging on the sofa. In spring, cardio exercise such as running, spinning, or HIIT help move through blockage and stagnation. Start to adapt your yoga practice to a stronger and more vigorous flow, such as Ashtanga and vinyasa-style yoga. Remember to stretch the sides of your body (ribs and IT band), where your liver and gallbladder meridian runs. Triangle pose *(trikonasana)*, side stretches, and gentle twists are great poses for spring. Also incorporate chest openers and backbends to move excess heaviness from the lungs and chest.

### *Green, Green, Greener*

Supporting yourself in spring can also be as simple as going for a walk in nature and taking in the vibrant green color that bursts forth in this season. Green nourishes both the liver and the wood element. That is why all the beautiful bitter greens (dandelion, nettles, arugula, chard, and spinach) are particularly cleansing for the liver and gallbladder and promote better digestion. When you are on your walk, try to move stuck energy by simply taking a few deep breaths (liver energy and Kapha tend to get stuck at the diaphragm and lungs). If you have an established breathing practice, you may experiment with switching your morning breathwork to more active, heating, and stimulating pranayama, such as skull-shining breath (*kapalabhati*) or bellows breath (*bhastrika*).

### *Brush Away Stagnation*

Stay warm and regularly visit a sauna to sweat and boost metabolism, lymph flow, and immunity. In spring, I also switch to dry-brushing before my abhyanga in the morning to boost lymphatic circulation. If you suffer from allergies, try tulsi tea or nettle tea in the spring, which both support lung and liver health.

## Summer: Recalibrate Your Pitta

June 21 marks the summer solstice—the longest day and shortest night of the year. It is the beginning of the summer season: hot days and balmy nights, time on the beach, joy, connection, playfulness, and celebration. In Ayurveda, it is the season of Pitta; and in Chinese medicine, the season of fire.

### *Summer Playfulness and Abundance*

During this time, yang energy is at its peak and with it light, warmth, and expansion. Summer bathes us in the physical and emotional warmth that comes with sun and fire. We enjoy long days, sun-kissed cheeks, and evenings spent outdoors under the stars with loved ones. Summer is playtime, and life flows easily and sweetly. Fire and Pitta are embodiments of the sun principle: They give life, energy, passion, and enthusiasm. Nature and life peak in summer and burst forth with an abundance of colors, flowers, sweet fruits, and juicy vegetables.

### *Cool Down*

As the weather starts heating up significantly, we do better to adjust our diet to summer, avoiding overly spicy and fried foods, heavy and heating red meat (lamb and beef), and fermented foods such as pickles and sauerkraut. Instead, we prefer using cooling oils, such as ghee or coconut oil, and cooling, nonspicy foods such as avocados, coconut, cucumbers, and juicy summer fruits such as melons. Summer is the time for beautiful salad bowls with plenty of fresh greens, crisp cucumbers, and nourishing avocados. With the increasing heat, our agni disperses and is weaker compared to winter. We naturally crave less and lighter foods, especially when the heat is strong. In summer, I try to do all my exercise early in the morning before sunrise, when the air is still cool and fresh. I adjust my yoga practice to be gentler and cooling, including forward bends, twists, and easy, nourishing inversions such as shoulder stand (*sarvangasana*). Swimming is my favorite exercise in summer. For those of you lucky enough to live near a lake or the ocean, make use of the cooling and soothing effect of water. My breathing practice will also change toward more cooling and gentler pranayama, such as alternate nostril breathing (*nadi shodhana*) and lunar breathing (*chandra bhedana*), especially when I feel overheated.

### *Try Moon Bathing*

Instead of excessive sunbathing, especially during the peak heat of the day between 11 a.m. and 4 p.m., I like to use the early morning and evening to be more playful outside and in the water. At night, especially around the full moon, you may also try the practice of "moon bathing." The moonlight's cooling, nourishing, yin-balancing properties are especially useful during the hot summer months when our body and mind tend to overheat and our mind feels restless and irritable. Moon bathing can be done at any phase of the moon, but the best healing properties are during full and new moon cycles. The full moon has stronger nourishing and yin-boosting juicy qualities, while the new moon has more cleansing and detoxifying properties. You can simply sit for fifteen to thirty minutes outside under the moon or by the window. You can also take a walk in the moonlight.

### *Use Coconut for Cooling*

You can also make a point in summer of wearing clothing with more cooling colors, such as white, gray, blue, and green; and avoiding warming colors, such as red, orange, dark yellow, and black. Drink plenty of room-temperature water or coconut water, a fantastic cooling and rehydrating beverage that is rich in electrolytes. For your daily abhyanga, I recommend using cooling coconut oil with a few drops of sandalwood and rose essential oils.

One of my favorite summer teas is an overnight cold infusion of rose petals, mint, and licorice. Remember, Ayurveda does not recommend iced drinks because they greatly suppress agni, but you could consume this tea at room temperature or lightly cooled.

# 5

## Hack 2: Transform

Harness Your Digestive and Metabolic Power

### Why Digestion and Metabolism Are Central: An Ayurvedic and Western Medicine Perspective

I praise Agni, the high priest of the sacrifice, the divine ministrant of the offering, who bestows upon us the treasures of life.
—*Rigveda* 1.1

Just as there would be no life on earth without the sun, there is no life in the body without agni, the Sanskrit word for "fire." In the Vedas, the oldest sacred texts of Hinduism, Agni is described as the god of fire and the messenger between the gods and humans.[1] It is Agni who carries the offerings of humans to the gods, and his flames are believed to purify these offerings and make them suitable for the gods to consume. We see Agni's representation in two forms: a celestial form that resides in the heavens (embodied by lightning and the sun), and an earthly form that burns in our kitchen stoves and (in India) in the form of a ghee lamp on many altars.

#### *Fire Is Consciousness and Transformation*

Out of all the elements, fire is the only one that transforms everything it encounters while itself not changing form. Therefore, traditionally in India, fire is associated with purity and transformation. Hindu priests and sadhus—ascetics who have renounced the world and dedicated their lives to spiritual pursuits—wear orange robes to symbolize the fire element and its association with consciousness, purity, and renunciation. Also, after death, Hindus cremate the body. By burning it to ash, they destroy any remaining impurities, release the soul from the physical body, and ultimately free it from the cycle of birth and death.

### *Health Is a Question of Fire*

In Ayurveda, too, health is a question of fire. If your internal fire burns strong and your digestion is flawless, you're dialed into longevity. A well-known Ayurvedic saying states that "you are as old as your agni," which means that your age is directly reflected in the strength and vitality of your digestive, metabolic, and mitochondrial power. Rather than chronological age, it is your biological age, measured according to certain biomarkers, that determines longevity. The ancient physicians knew what modern science is only now beginning to fully discover: One of the most important factors in overall health is the state of your digestive and metabolic power—agni.

### *An Ayurvedic Perspective on Digestion*

How well you digest, assimilate, absorb, and metabolize not only food but also information, thoughts, emotions, and experiences all depends on the state and strength of your internal fire. There are countless agnis in the body, since all metabolic functions are governed by fire, but the main agni is the *jathara agni,* the digestive fire that sits in the stomach and small intestine. Jathara agni is the main gate through which nutrients enter the tissues and then pass on to individual cells. It includes gastric mucous secretions, hunger regulation in the brain, peristalsis, and various gastric and intestinal enzymes. After jathara agni in the stomach breaks down the food, it progresses to the small intestines where it is absorbed by villi into the hepatic circulatory system. In the liver, the broken-down food molecules are worked on by the *bhuta agnis* (elemental fires), which transform the five elements of food (space, air, fire, water, earth) into five biologically available elements that are then circulated to the individual *dhatus* (tissues) for nourishment.

## How to Transform: You Are What You Digest—Agni and Ama

You all have heard the saying "You are what you eat." According to Ayurveda, it actually is "You are what you digest" because your agni, or digestive power, is what makes or breaks you. Health starts with proper digestion, and disease starts with impaired digestion. Why? Because weak digestion results in the accumulation of toxins, or ama, which then start clogging the channels and lead to tissue inflammation. We will discuss ama in a moment, but for now remember that impaired digestion is the precursor to almost every chronic disease.

When looking at the various nutritional guidelines that Ayurveda puts forth, it is helpful to remind ourselves of the intrinsic link between macro and micro. I find it extremely helpful to compare our internal digestion to the external preparation or cooking of food.

**Digestive Analogy**

Pot = Stomach

Food = Today's meal

Water = (*Kledaka*) Kapha, a subtype of Kapha that resides in the stomach

Agni = (*Pachaka*) Pitta, a subtype of Pitta that resides in the stomach and small intestine

Fireplace = Small intestine

Air = (*Samana*) Vayu, a subtype of Vata that resides in the small intestine

Fuel = Yesterday's digested food

According to this analogy, it makes complete sense that Ayurveda recommends certain food practices to support optimal digestion. I will go into details later, but for now I just want to give a few examples.

### *The Logic Behind Ayurveda's Dietary Rules*

Just like the flame on your stove, agni, the digestive fire, is hot, light, sharp, penetrating, pungent, and clear. This is why cold food is generally not recommended in Ayurveda: Our agni requires heat for biotransformation. Similarly, Ayurveda does not recommend drinking large amounts of (cold) water with meals. Just like you would not cook a pot of rice while continuously adding more and more water, you cannot properly digest if you dilute your digestive enzymes by drinking too many fluids with meals, even more so if they are cold. Ayurveda also does not recommend frequent snacking or eating before the previous meal has been digested (at least four hours). This is very similar to cooking rice and every ten minutes adding more rice. This will result in some of the rice being overcooked, while some won't be cooked at all. It is the same in our digestive system. Snacking or eating before the previous meal has been digested leads to indigestion, gas, bloating, and ama (endotoxins).

### How to Optimize Digestion

**Regularity:** Eat at regular times and avoid snacking between meals.

**Luxurious lunch:** Make lunch your biggest meal, and make dinner early and light.

**Healthy hunger:** Eat only when hungry, which means your previous meal has been fully digested. Fast at least twelve to fourteen hours overnight.

**Time your liquids:** Don't drink large amounts of (cold) water with meals, but make sure to drink a large glass of water one hour before a meal to ensure there are enough fluids available for proper stomach acid and digestive enzyme production.

**Spice it up:** Use digestive spices such as ginger, cumin, coriander, or cinnamon.

### *Perfect Digestion*

When agni is balanced, then digestion, absorption, and elimination are all normal. You can digest any type of food in any season without adverse signs and symptoms. We call this *sama agni*, or balanced agni. Sama agni guarantees excellent health, strong immunity, and longevity. It also encourages positive emotional states such as courage, optimism, and brightness. Our constitution often (but not always) predisposes us to certain digestive imbalances, collectively known as our digestive dosha, which of course can change according to the seasons or our eating habits.

## How Strong Is Your Digestive Power? Check Your Agni Dosha

Here is a quick assessment tool for checking your general digestive and metabolic tendencies, your so-called agni dosha. I suggest two rounds. For now, please answer only according to your *general* tendencies when you look over your lifetime. Later, when we determine your imbalances before you set out to embark on your Ayurveda 2.0 journey, you can answer according to your *current* digestive symptoms.

1. How do you usually feel after eating a meal?
   a. I feel satiated and full of energy.
   b. I often feel bloated or gassy.
   c. Usually good. But if I eat foods that are too spicy or oily, I can get heartburn, acidity, or reflux.
   d. I can easily feel heavy, stuffed, and sleepy after meals. My energy goes down.

2. How is your appetite and hunger level?
   a. Pretty regular.
   b. My appetite varies every day. If I am busy, I forget to eat. Often my eyes are bigger than my stomach.
   c. My appetite is strong. I am almost always hungry and can eat big portions.
   d. My appetite is low. I can feel full for a long time after eating. I eat more for pleasure and comfort than actual hunger.

3. What happens if you skip a meal?
   a. I can easily skip a meal and feel totally fine.
   b. I need to eat more frequently. If I forget to eat, I can easily get lightheaded and hypoglycemic.

c. I hate skipping meals. I get cranky, irritable, and (h)angry.
d. I can easily skip meals and feel much better if I eat less.

4. Which foods tend to bother you the most?
   a. I can usually eat everything and digest it well.
   b. I usually get gassy and bloated with raw salads; beans and lentils; and cruciferous vegetables such as broccoli, cabbage, and cauliflower.
   c. If I eat fried, oily, or spicy foods, I can get heartburn and acid reflux.
   d. I tend to get sleepy and/or congested after eating sweets, refined carbs, and dairy products such as cheese, yogurt, or ice cream.

5. How is your elimination?
   a. Normal. I have a well-formed bowel movement every morning.
   b. Irregular. I often have constipation with dry and small pellet stools.
   c. Frequent. I can have two to three bowel movements per day, often on the soft or liquid side.
   d. Regular. My stools are generally heavy and bulky. Rarely, there also can be mucous in the stool.

Now count how many a, b, c, and d answers you got. It is possible that you scored high in one or two categories. This is your agni dosha, your general digestive capacity and tendency for imbalances. Agni has four clinical states:

a. *Sama* (balanced)
b. *Vishama* (irregular)
c. *Tikshna* (sharp and acidic)
d. *Manda* (dull and slow)

Ideally we want to be as close to sama agni (balanced digestion) as possible, since this is the only true healthy state of agni. But often constitutionally we tend toward one of the other forms of pathological agni.

## Results

### *a. Balanced Digestion (Sama Agni)*

If you scored mostly **a** answers, you have sama agni, which is a balanced digestive system. Your digestion, absorption, and elimination are all normal, and you can digest any type of food in any season without adverse signs and symptoms.

### *b. Irregular Digestion (Vishama Agni)*

If you scored mostly **b** answers, you have vishama agni, which is a Mover digestive system. Movers tend toward weak and irregular digestion and dry, infrequent elimination. Agni can fluctuate and become erratic, producing irregular appetite, variable digestion, bloating, gas, constipation, and colicky pain. If not corrected, over time this can lead to degenerative Vata disorders such as arthritis, osteoporosis, insomnia, and even Parkinson's and MS.

**Remedy: Regularity and Routine.** People with vishama agni need a proper eating routine and regular mealtimes to stabilize their fickle and changing agni. Movers generally love grazing and snacking, but their digestive fire functions better with three substantial meals that can be smaller and more frequent. Meals for Movers should always include complex carbohydrates such as sweet potatoes or quinoa, and enough (animal) protein and healthy fats to keep them nourished and sustained. This stabilizes their blood sugar and prevents energy crashes and hypoglycemia.

### *c. Acidic Digestion (Tikshna Agni)*

If you scored mostly **c** answers, you have tikshna agni, which is a Transformer digestive system. Transformers can develop an irritated, inflamed, and acidic digestive system. Here, agni can become intense and cause craving for large quantities of food. After eating, one gets a dry throat and lips as well as heartburn and acid reflux or diarrhea. There also may be intense craving for sweets. Over time, inflammatory

Pitta disorders such as gastritis, acne or psoriasis, colitis, or autoimmune conditions can develop.

**Remedy: No Fried, Acidic, or Spicy Foods.** People with tikshna agni burn through food faster than others. They need timely and regular meals to prevent becoming (h)angry or developing acidity. They usually do well with two to three solid meals per day. Avoiding spicy and oily foods as well as too much coffee and alcohol will help prevent tikshna agni disorders such as heartburn and reflux, or down-the-line chronic inflammatory bowel disorders such as Crohn's disease or ulcerative colitis.

*d. Slow Digestion (Manda Agni)*

If you scored mostly **d** answers, you have manda agni, which is a Regenerator digestive system. Regenerators are prone to dull, slow, and sluggish digestion and metabolism. Even when fasting, a person with manda agni can put on weight. There is heaviness in the stomach, loss of appetite, fullness, and sleepiness after meals. Over time it can lead to congestive Kapha disorders such as allergies, edema, fibroids, cysts, and tumors.

**Remedy: Eat Light and Space Out Meals.** People with manda agni digest food the slowest and do great on intermittent fasting (IF), with a fasting window of at least sixteen hours. They feel best with one or two meals a day, a late brunch and/or early dinner. If they overeat or eat before their meal has been properly digested (at least six hours after a meal), they are likely to experience heaviness, brain fog, indigestion, and weight gain.

## Powerful Agni Hacks

### Before Meals

- Chew a slice of Ayurvedic Ginger Pickle (see page 226).
- Take one tablespoon of apple cider vinegar with a little warm water. This supports healthy stomach acid and balances your blood sugar levels after meals.

- Before you start eating, take a few deep breaths to center. Acknowledge gratitude that you have food on your plate that gives strength, nourishment, and sustenance.

### During Meals

- Don't drink large amounts of (cold) water with your meals.
- Eat slowly, mindfully, and joyfully.
- Don't multitask, work, or discuss sensitive or problematic subjects while eating.

### After Meals

- Take a leisurely walk or lie on your left side for five minutes. Both support proper digestion.
- Chew a half teaspoon of Happy Belly Spice (see page 228) to enhance absorption and prevent gas and bloating after meals.
- Drink a cup of Tame the Flame Tea (see page 226), one of the best tonics for proper digestion and absorption.

## Ama—Toxicity

If agni is your hero, then ama is the villain. When agni is impaired, mostly through detrimental lifestyle choices such as skipping meals or eating on the go, wrong food combinations, overeating, or repressed emotions, then the food we eat does not get fully digested and a toxic residue (*ama*) is created.

### *Ama Is at the Root of Most Disease*

*Ama* literally translates as "unripe" or "uncooked" and refers to this internally-generated metabolic waste (endotoxins). To some degree, the formation of small amounts of ama is a normal part of the digestive process because until your food is fully digested, which takes between three to six hours, it is ama, or "uncooked." But if ama starts to build up in the gut due to unsuitable dietary habits and chronic indigestion, it causes inflammation and micro-tearing in the delicate mucosal lining of the small intestine. Once compromised, the gut membranes become permeable (often referred to as "leaky gut syndrome"), and food particles escape from the digestive tract into the bloodstream, where they trigger the immune system and initiate inflammation throughout the entire body. The result is chronic fatigue, weight gain, brain fog, mood disorders, and often eventually autoimmune disease.[2]

### *Cellular Dysfunction*

Furthermore, when ama is generated in large amounts, the toxic load becomes too high for the body to handle and cannot be properly cleared and eliminated. Once ama spreads into circulation, accumulates, and eventually deposits in the deeper tissues, it starts clogging the channels, disrupts tissue nutrition and waste removal, and coats individual cell membranes. Eventually this leads to a loss of cellular intelligence and compromised cellular function and signaling. This is why Ayurveda considers ama to be at the root of most diseases and has developed elaborate detoxification therapies that systematically remove deep-seated ama from the body tissues (*panchakarma*).

#### WHAT CAUSES AMA?

- Overeating or frequent snacking before the previous meal is digested
- Eating heavy, oily, or deep-fried foods
- Eating leftovers (food that has been sitting outside or in the fridge for longer than six hours)
- Choosing cold and heavy-to-digest foods such as ice cream, cheese, or cold milkshakes
- Eating dinner late
- Snacking after dinner, before bed, or late at night
- Keeping irregular eating habits
- Relying heavily on processed and packaged foods
- Eating out frequently, especially fast foods
- Choosing incompatible food combinations
- Engaging in emotional (over)eating or binging

*Note: Ayurveda and Leftovers*

One of the most important tenants of Ayurvedic nutrition—and one that is not always easy to follow—is to eat freshly cooked foods. This means avoiding leftovers, which strictly speaking is anything that is cooked and left for longer than four to six hours. Food that is leftover, frozen, or reheated is considered lacking life force (prana). Also, especially when keeping food overnight (or several days) in the refrigerator, it starts decomposing; it becomes cold and clogging to the channels, which lowers agni and generates ama (endotoxins).

When I first started practicing in Turkey, this was probably the most difficult suggestion for people to follow because traditionally in Turkish cooking, large amounts of *zeytinyağlılar* (traditional olive oil dishes) are prepared, stored in the fridge, and eaten for several days. I have many Turkish friends who claim the food tastes better on the second or third day. While for most of us living busy lives—and often juggling work, family, and social obligations—it can feel daunting to cook every meal from scratch, we can at least attempt to cook as fresh as possible and in smaller portions, and store leftover food for a maximum of one day and not more. Often it is just a matter of good planning and prioritizing that allows us to cook fresh most of the time.

## Assess Your Level of Ama

To assess if you have ama as a result of imbalanced eating habits and poor digestion, please check the list below and mark each symptom that applies to you.

- ❒ Lack of appetite and taste
- ❒ Bad breath
- ❒ Thick tongue coating
- ❒ Smelly gas and stools
- ❒ Sticky stools that stain the toilet
- ❒ Indigestion
- ❒ Chronic mucous or congestion
- ❒ Feeling of heaviness and lethargy
- ❒ Brain fog

- ☐ Smelly sweat and/or urine
- ☐ Joint inflammation and pain
- ☐ Dull aches and pains (especially whole body and roots of hair)
- ☐ Skin issues such as acne, pimples, rashes

Total: ____________________

< 2 Bravo. Your level of toxicity is zero or very low and mostly limited to your digestive system.

2–3 There is some level of ama in your digestive system and possibly also in systemic circulation.

> 3 You have ama in your digestive system, systemic circulation, and possibly even lodged in the deeper tissues.

If you have marked more than one symptom on the list above, it is likely that you have some ama in your system. More than three checkmarks means your body is in need of some cleansing and a digestive reboot.

## Your Metabolic Type and Ama

Let's briefly look at what happens when ama starts amalgamating or mixing with the doshas.

### *Movers: Toxins Accumulate in Colon, Joints, and Bones*

In Movers, ama tends to accumulate in the lower abdomen and pelvis, causing bloating, constipation, cramps, and pain. If left untreated, ama can start lodging in body parts where Vata is already dominant, such as the colon, brain, and bones, and lead to more serious disorders such as diverticulitis, arthritis, or neurodegenerative diseases.

### *Transformers: Toxins Accumulate in the Small Intestine, Blood, and Skin*

In Transformers, ama tends to accumulate in the center of the body around the belly button, and causes inflammation in the small intestine, liver, and gallbladder, as well as toxicity in the blood. It can create a bitter or metallic taste in the mouth, heartburn or acid reflux, diarrhea, and skin diseases. Left untreated, it can cause more serious disorders such as ulcers or inflammatory bowel disorders (Crohn's disease, colitis), skin disorders, and widespread inflammation and autoimmune conditions.

### *Regenerators: Toxins Accumulate in the Chest and Lymph*

In Regenerators, ama tends to accumulate in the stomach, chest, and sinuses, where it causes low appetite and lethargy, as well as mucous and congestion. Left untreated, it can further congest the lymph tissue, leading to metabolic disorders, obesity, cysts or fibroids, diabetes, and high cholesterol or triglycerides.

## Two Simple Tricks to Prevent and Treat Ama: Fasting and Hot Water

It may sound strange, but the top two remedies for built-up ama are deceptively simple and cheap. They require no expensive pills, supplements, or gadgets. The first trick is fasting. Fasting gives your agni the chance to "digest" ama instead of working on your pizza. The second trick is sipping on hot water, also called *garam pani* in India. Hot water is a superfood. It cleanses and hydrates the digestive tract, stimulates the lymphatic system, and strengthens agni. Hot water also vasodilates the channels (*srotamsi*), supporting circulation and promoting elimination of wastes and cellular ama. Just think about washing dishes or a dirty piece of clothing with cold water versus hot water. Hot water is much more efficient.

### *How to Do It: Fasting*

With fasting, you can refer to the following chapter on lymph and fasting to determine what type of fasting is most suitable for you. Very simply, however, it may mean just skipping breakfast after having a heavy dinner the night before or skipping dinner after a heavier lunch. This gives agni the chance to deal with the backlog of food.

### *How to Do It: Hot Water Therapy*

For hot water therapy, ideally you boil water in a glass or stainless-steel pot uncovered for at least ten minutes. This subtly changes the properties and molecules of the water, making it easier to assimilate. If this is not possible or practical, use regular boiled water and sip on it every thirty minutes between meals.

### *If You Need Deeper Cleansing*

When we need a little deeper cleansing, then pungent and bitter herbs and spices are called for, many of which you already have in your kitchen. Pungent spices such as ginger, cumin, black pepper, asafetida/hing, fennel, and cinnamon are fantastic "ama burners" for Movers and Regenerators, while more neutral and slightly bitter spices such as cumin, coriander, and fennel seeds are better for Transformers. Bitter herbs such as gentian, neem, and guggulu are also very useful for ama, especially for Transformers and Regenerators. Finally, fresh or dried turmeric root can and should be used by all types since it is a superb anti-inflammatory, ama-reducing, and gut-flora-rebuilding spice. Also remember, when there is too much ama, fast or eat only light and warm foods (broths and soups) to give your digestion time to recuperate and burn through the backlog of ama instead of having to digest your current meal.

### *Balancing Vata (Mover) Ama*

Because Vata ama tends to accumulate specifically in the large intestine, fiber and mild laxatives or bowel lubricants (demulcents) can be extremely helpful. Psyllium husk, Triphala powder, aloe vera gel, or the occasional spoon of castor oil at bedtime all help to remove Vata ama from the colon. Tame the Flame Spice, classically called Hingvasthak Churna (see page 227), is also helpful when taken at a dose of a half teaspoon directly on the tongue, sprinkled over food, or with a little ghee after meals.

### *Balancing Pitta (Transformer) Ama*

Pitta ama responds well to stronger purgation and bitter herbs. A classical formula used in India is *avipatti* powder or *trivrit leham* (paste) taken with warm water at bedtime. You can also use the Western herb rhubarb root as an occasional purgative. Additional bitter herbs to include are coriander seeds and leaf, neem leaf, and turmeric root.

### *Balancing Kapha (Regenerator) Ama*

Because Kapha ama concentrates in the stomach, lungs, and lymph, it responds well to herbs and spices that are pungent, bitter, and astringent. Especially Fire Up Spice, classically called trikatu churna (see page 227)—a potent mix of dry ginger, black pepper, and Indian long pepper (*pippali*) powders—kick-starts agni and clears ama as well as excessive mucous. Sprinkle it on food or take a quarter teaspoon on the tongue before meals. In case of cold, congestion, or mucous, mix the powders with honey and lick a half teaspoon every three to four hours followed by sipping a half cup of hot water.

## Ancient Functional Nutrition: Beyond Fats, Carbs, and Proteins

In Ayurveda, eating according to your constitution and season, along with a routine that enhances digestion, is considered the best medicine and highly supportive of agni. Rather than focusing on macronutrients such as proteins, carbohydrates, and fats, Ayurveda approaches food energetically, considering the elemental composition, its qualities (*gunas*), and tastes (*rasas*).

### *Elements and Food*

One way to classify foods in Ayurveda is according to the elements. Remember, elements are not abstract concepts but functional aspects of all substances. The framework of elements is extremely useful if you know that your constitution is deficient or aggravated in a particular element, or if you are living in a climate where a certain element is strongly dominating. Examples would be a dominant water element in the tropics, such as Hawaii, or cold and wet places such as London; or excessive air and space elements in high-desert climates like New Mexico.

**Earth:** Foods dominant in the earth element are generally grounding, nourishing, and building. They include nuts and seeds, beans, grains, mushrooms, root vegetables, and animal proteins such as eggs, fish, and meat.

**Water:** Foods dominant in the water element are nourishing and cooling and help to lubricate the tissues and replenish bodily fluids. They include milk and dairy products; juicy fruits such as grapes, melon, and peaches; and juicy vegetables such as cucumbers, tomatoes, and zucchini.

**Fire:** Foods dominant in the fire element usually help to increase agni, warm the body, and eliminate toxicity. They include most (pungent) spices such as black pepper, chili, cinnamon, cloves, and ginger; sour fruits such as grapefruit, lemon, and pineapple; and heating and inflammatory substances like alcohol, coffee, and cigarettes.

**Air:** Foods dominant in the air element can cause gas and bloating if consumed in excess or not properly prepared. These include all dried fruits; raw vegetables, sprouts, and salads; cruciferous vegetables such as broccoli, cabbage, and cauliflower; and legumes such as beans and lentils.

**Ether:** This is not such an easy category to comprehend. The ether element's dominant qualities are subtle and clear, so ether-predominant foods are known for their strong cleansing action. Foods dominant in the ether element include wheatgrass or fresh (green) vegetable juices, as well as microalgae such as chlorella and spirulina. (Recreational) drugs, cigarettes, coffee, and alcohol also all have an ether component since they strongly, quickly, and directly affect the mind due to their subtle quality.

### *Radically Rethinking Nutritional Science: Qualities (Gunas) of Foods*

One of the most important features of the Ayurvedic nutritional model is the concept of *gunas* (qualities) of food. In Ayurveda, what quality a particular food has is more important than its nutritional content because gunas are what directly influence the doshas in the body and mind. You may remember the twenty gunas from chapter 2. For simplicity's sake, instead of focusing on all twenty, when it comes to Ayurvedic nutrition, we usually consider the three most important pairs.

**Master the Six Gunas**

| | |
|---|---|
| Hot | Cold |
| Heavy | Light |
| Dry | Moist/Oily |

Examples of the hot or heating quality are all spices, sour fruits, pungent vegetables (garlic, onion, radishes), red meat (beef, lamb), and alcohol. Cooling foods include coconut, cucumbers, juicy fruits such as melons, and milk. Examples of dry foods are dried fruits, crackers, bread, legumes, and grains such as buckwheat or polenta. Moist or oily foods include dairy products, ghee, oils, nuts, juicy vegetables, and juicy fruits. Light foods include popcorn, sprouts, crackers, berries, and greens; whereas heavy foods include meat, beans, nuts, and grains, especially wheat.

### *Heavier and Nourishing Foods for Vata*

Working with these six gunas is quite simple. Remember, we always balance through opposites. Because Vata is cold, dry, and light, foods that are warming, moist or oily, and heavy (earth-element dominant) are wonderfully balancing. This could be oily nuts and seeds; earthy root vegetables and mushrooms; heavier and moistening grains such as oats or wheat; sweet fruits such as grapes, figs, or peaches; and warming spices such as cinnamon and ginger.

### *Cooling Foods for Pitta*

Similarly, Pitta is hot, oily, and light, so foods that are cooling, dry, or heavy are balancing. Leafy greens, sprouts, fresh cucumbers, juicy summer fruits such as apricots and peaches, drier grains such as basmati rice and millet, and cooling or neutral spices such as coriander and mint are all balancing.

### *Light and Stimulating Foods for Kapha*

Because Kapha is cold, heavy, and moist or oily, we balance it through warming, light, and dry foods. We can choose vegetables higher in the air element such as broccoli, cabbage, and cauliflower; warming, drier grains such as buckwheat and corn; astringent fruits such as berries and pomegranates; and stronger spices that kick-start metabolism, such as dried ginger, black pepper, cloves, and chili.

## The Six Tastes (*Shad Rasa*)

According to Ayurvedic wisdom, just as important as the qualities of a food are the tastes. While in the West we have traditionally only identified five tastes (sweet, sour, salty, bitter, and umami), Ayurveda holds that there are six tastes: *madhura* (sweet), *amla* (sour), *lavana* (salty), *tikta* (bitter), *katu* (pungent), and *kashaya* (astringent).

### *Digestion Starts on Your Tongue*

The six tastes are fundamental for digestion. This is because each taste has a certain elemental composition, which has a direct influence on the body, the organs, and the doshas. Also, digestion begins the moment you put food in your mouth and your tongue picks up the tastes of your food. Located on your tongue are thousands of taste buds that each contain between fifty to one hundred taste receptor cells. These are responsible for perceiving taste and sending signals to the brain to prime the gut to start secreting the right enzymes to be able to digest and assimilate the incoming food.[3] So just by tasting a food, your body knows how to handle it. This is why in Ayurveda we usually prefer giving herbs in liquid or powder form rather than capsules. That way their taste is directly communicated to the body, and they are better absorbed and assimilated, and thus, also more potent and effective.

### *Taste Receptors Are Not Only in Your Mouth*

In the past decade, science has discovered that taste receptor cells are not only confined to the oral cavity. Even some of your organs, such as the gut and pancreas, have taste receptor cells. Rather than conveying the sensation of taste to the brain, activation of these receptor cells triggers the release of hormones that regulate appetite, satiety, and metabolic processes.[4]

According to Ayurveda, a balanced diet should always contain all six tastes. Today in the West, most processed diets, however, favor the addictive sweet and salty tastes by far and are greatly lacking the other tastes.

### *Sweet Taste: Builds and Nourishes*

The sweet taste comprises the earth and water elements, and its qualities are cooling and heavy. The bulk of foods we consume daily are part of this category since it is the most basic and building taste. Examples are, of course, sweeteners such as sugar or honey and fruits. But grains, sweet root vegetables, dairy products such as milk and fresh unfermented cheese, and meat are also considered sweet due to their elemental composition.

**The Best Taste to Sustain Health Is Sweet.** In Ayurveda, we say that sweet is the best taste for someone who is healthy, while bitter is the best taste for someone who is sick. Here is why: In moderation, the sweet taste is wholesome to the body, promoting healthy growth of all bodily tissues and increasing strength and vitality. It balances both Vata and Pitta doshas and is considered nourishing and regenerative. The bulk of our food—fruits, grains, root vegetables, meat, milk, nuts—falls under the sweet taste because it is the most important taste for rejuvenation and homeostasis. Refined sugar and carbohydrates, however, as well as overuse of sweet, aggravates Kapha dosha and compromises lungs, thyroid, and pancreas, causing cold, congestion, heaviness, loss of appetite, dysbiosis and fungal or parasitic infections, metabolic syndrome (obesity), and diabetes.

### *Sour Taste: Refreshes and Stimulates Digestion*

The sour taste comprises the earth and fire elements, and its qualities are liquid, light, and heating. Examples include citrus fruits, vinegar, and tomato, as well as all fermented foods such as kefir, kimchi, sauerkraut, and yogurt. Used in moderation, the sour taste is refreshing, stimulates appetite, improves digestion, energizes the body, and brightens the mind. It balances Vata dosha. Used in excess, however, it aggravates Pitta and Kapha, causing inflammation, hyperacidity, heartburn, and ulcers.

### *Salty Taste: Improves Taste and Supports Adrenals*

The salty taste comprises the water and fire elements, and its qualities are heating, heavy, oily, and hydrophilic (attracting water). The organs directly affected by the salty taste are the kidneys and adrenals, which is why we often crave salty foods (chips, salty fries or nuts) when we are stressed or our adrenals are depleted. Examples of the salty taste are obvious: sea and pink salt, kelp, seaweeds, and (saltwater) fish. Used moderately, the salty taste relieves Vata. Like the sweet and sour tastes, it is anabolic (tissue-building), improves the flavor of food, and aids digestion, absorption, and the elimination of wastes. Excessive salt intake, however, can aggravate Pitta and Kapha, and is said to thicken the blood and cause hypertension, as well as contribute to early wrinkles and baldness. Owing to its hydrophilic nature, it may also lead to water retention, congestion, and edema.

### *Pungent Taste: Ignites Digestion*

Probably the most potent taste of all, the pungent taste is made up of the fire and air elements, and has light, drying, and heating qualities. It directly affects the stomach and intestines, as well as the heart. Examples of the pungent taste include chili, garlic, ginger, mustard, onion, and radish. Used in moderation, pungency can fire up agni, aid digestion and absorption, clear sinuses and mucous, increase circulation, and break up stagnation. While it is balancing to Kapha (and in small amounts to Vata), when overused, the pungent taste vitiates both Pitta and Vata, causing burning, sweating, ulcers, hypertension, dryness, sexual debility, and infertility.

### *Bitter Taste: Detoxifying and Anti-Inflammatory*

The bitter taste comprises the air and ether elements, and the qualities are cool, light, and drying. It directly affects the pancreas, spleen, liver, and gallbladder. Examples of the bitter taste are turmeric, neem, fenugreek, arugula, dandelion, turmeric, and coffee. As I mentioned earlier, while sweet is considered the best taste for healthy people, in disease the bitter taste is preferred because it is highly detoxifying, as well as antibacterial, antifungal, and anti-inflammatory. Many herbal medicines in fact are bitter, such as artichoke leaves, dandelion, gentian, neem, nettles, and turmeric. The bitter taste pacifies Pitta and Kapha, reduces fever, and stimulates firmness of skin and muscles. It is also anti-toxic and kills germs. As it is severely drying to the system, chronic overuse can aggravate Vata and cause depletion in body fat and bone marrow, extreme dryness, weight loss, and weakness.

### *Astringent Taste: Reduces Edema and Firms Tissues*

Comprising the air and earth elements, the qualities of the astringent taste are cooling and drying. The taste directly affects the colon. Examples include unripe or green bananas, legumes, pomegranates, and turmeric. In moderation, it balances Pitta and Kapha, reduces dampness and water retention, and tightens skin and muscles. Excessive use aggravates Vata, causing constipation, stagnation of circulation, and spasms; long-term overuse can lead to emaciation and neuromuscular Vata disorders.

Movers are balanced by the sweet, sour, and salty tastes; and aggravated by the pungent, bitter, and astringent tastes.

Transformers are balanced by the sweet, bitter, and astringent tastes; and aggravated by the pungent, sour, and salty tastes.

Regenerators are balanced by the bitter, pungent, and astringent tastes and aggravated by sweet, sour, salty tastes.

### *Potency (Virya)*

The potency of a food is about its effect on our metabolism, no matter what its temperature is at the time of consumption. For example, a cold glass of red wine still has a heating effect on the body, while a hot mint tea has a cooling action. In general, heating foods increase metabolism and promote weight loss; cooling foods slow down metabolism and promote weight gain and rejuvenation.

Foods with a heating potency (chili, citrus, garlic, ginger, mustard) pacify Vata and Kapha but can stimulate Pitta. They promote digestion and metabolism, kindle agni, increase body temperature, and enhance circulation. If used excessively, they can cause tikshna agni (sharp hypermetabolism), hypoglycemia, gastritis, ulcers, and inflammation.

Foods with a cooling potency (avocados, coconut, cucumbers, dairy, salads) pacify Pitta but can stimulate Vata and Kapha. They promote anabolic activity (growth and rejuvenation), slow down agni, and relieve burning, irritation, and inflammation. If used excessively, they can create manda agni (dull hypometabolism), abnormal growths and cysts, slow metabolism, obesity and poor digestion, malabsorption, and ama (endotoxicity).

## Undiet: Tailored Foods for Movers (Vata), Transformers (Pitta), Regenerators (Kapha)

In Ayurveda, no two people are alike, and what might work for your digestion and metabolism might be detrimental for someone else. This is why there is not one diet that fits all. We are made to believe that whatever diet trend is circulating—be it low fat, low carb, keto, paleo, veganism, or raw food—is the solution for everybody's digestive and weight problems. The truth is that these diets work very well for some people but not for others.

### *We Naturally Cycle Through Diets During the Year*

Usually when there is a lot of media noise, hype, and confusion about health and nutrition, I like to go back to the basics and look to time-tested, ancient, nutritional models that are based on concepts such as bio-individuality and seasonality. As the Ayurvedic physician John Douillard explained in his beautiful book *The 3-Season Diet*, we are naturally shifting our diet with the seasons. In winter, for example, our body is programmed to build and store energy, so our diet—in line with the harvest of the fall and winter season—is naturally heavier—that is, more root vegetables, meat stews, nuts, and seeds. In spring, when the winter storages run low and nature has not yet started giving an abundant harvest, we traditionally fast and eat a Kapha-reducing, low-fat, plant-based diet. Nature provides all the beautiful cleansing bitter roots and greens (such as artichokes, dandelion, and nettles) to detoxify the liver and gallbladder from the heavier diet of winter. In many cultural and religious traditions, this is the time to fast and cleanse the body from the sluggishness of the winter season. Summer, on the other hand, offers a bounty of juicy, ripe fruits and vegetables, and we naturally follow more of a cooling and energy-sustaining high-carb diet. You see, even throughout the year, our diet shifts from high-protein and high-fat (winter) to vegan and low-fat (spring) and more raw foods and high-carb (summer), naturally with the rhythm of the seasons.

## Mover (Vata) or Fall and Early-Winter Diet

We have seen that Movers' digestive tendency is toward irregular appetite and elimination, indigestion, gas and bloating, and constipation. Usually fall and early winter (October–January) is the most challenging time for Mover types; and bloating, lower back pain, dryness, and irregular appetite with constipation is not uncommon during this season. Since some of the qualities of Vata are cold, light, and dry, they do best with warm, heavy, and moist foods as well as the sweet, sour, and salty tastes.

### *Warm, Cooked, and Nourishing Meals*

In general, Movers (or everybody during Vata season) should prefer cooked, warm, soupy foods rather than cold sandwiches and raw salads. Well-cooked, moist, and building grains (basmati rice, oats, quinoa) and grounding root vegetables (beets, carrots, pumpkin, sweet potatoes) all help support Movers by nourishing and grounding their restless body and mind. Smaller beans such as red or yellow lentils and mung beans (well soaked for at least twelve hours) are easier for Movers to digest than larger white beans and chickpeas. Dairy is usually fine, especially warm milk with digestive spices such as cinnamon or cardamom; and kefir and fresh cheese, such as mozzarella or goat cheese. Sweet juicy fruits (fresh figs, sweet grapes, oranges) are better than astringent and airy fruits (apples, pomegranates). Out of all constitutions, Movers do best with small amounts of animal protein such as eggs, bone broth, oily fish (sardines, wild salmon), and darker, oilier meats (beef, chicken legs, lamb, liver), always in small amounts, slow-cooked and well spiced for optimal digestion.

#### Mover Foods

Balancing tastes: sweet, sour, salty

Balancing gunas: warm, heavy, moist

Fruit: apricots, avocados, bananas, berries, cherries, dates, figs, grapefruits, grapes, kiwi, lemons, melons, oranges, peaches, plums, strawberries. Sweet or sour fruits are balancing.

Vegetables: asparagus, beets, carrots, cucumber, fennel, green beans, leeks, mustard greens, okra, olives, onion, parsnip, peas, potato (sweet), pumpkin, purslane, spinach, squash, watercress, zucchini. Cooked vegetables are most balancing. Avoid raw vegetables, especially in fall and winter.

Grains: basmati rice, oats, quinoa; ancient wheat types such as einkorn, emmer, or spelt

Legumes: mung beans; red, yellow, and green lentils; tempeh; and tofu

Dairy: butter, fresh cheese (ricotta, mozzarella), kefir, ghee, milk, yogurt

Nuts and seeds: almonds, Brazil nuts, cashews, chia seeds, flaxseeds, hazelnuts, hempseeds, pecan nuts, pine nuts, pistachios, pumpkin seeds, macadamia nuts, sesame seeds, sunflower seeds, walnuts

Oils: butter, coconut, ghee, hemp, olive or pumpkin-seed oil (always unrefined and cold-pressed)

Animal protein: eggs, beef, chicken, duck, oily fish (anchovies, sardines, bonito, wild-caught salmon), lamb, and turkey (dark meat)

Sweeteners: coconut sugar, date syrup, honey, maple syrup, or molasses

Spices: basil, bay leaf, cardamom, cinnamon, cloves, coriander, cumin, dill, fennel, ginger, nutmeg, oregano, parsley, rosemary, thyme

Drinks: almond, hemp, oat, or rice milk (warm and well spiced); chai, dandelion "coffee"; white tea; herbal teas (chamomile, fennel, ginger, honeybush, lemon balm, oat straw, rooibos, tulsi); full-bodied red wine

## Transformer (Pitta) or Summer Diet

Transformers usually have a strong digestion, good appetite, and desire for large quantities of food but can tend toward acidity, reflux, indigestion, and loose stools. Especially the summer months—June until September—can provoke excess fire in the body. Since the qualities of Pitta are hot, light, and oily during the summer months, Transformers do best with foods that are cooling and less oily, and the sweet, bitter, and astringent tastes.

### *Cooling Greens and Alkalinizing Grains*

In general, Transformers should stick to cooling and alkalinizing grains (barley, basmati rice, millet, oats, quinoa) and anti-inflammatory, blood-cleansing leafy green vegetables (arugula, chard, kale, nettles, spinach). Also fine for Pitta are sweet, juicy fruits (melons, nectarines, peaches), cooling oils (coconut oil, ghee), and fresh dairy (mozzarella, ricotta cheese). In terms of animal protein, white meats such as chicken or turkey breast and freshwater fish such as trout, which is more cooling, are more suitable.

### Transformer Foods

Balancing tastes: sweet, bitter, astringent

Balancing gunas: cool, heavy, dry

Fruit: apples, apricots, avocado, berries, cherries, dates, figs, grapes, melons, pears, plums, pomegranates, watermelon. Sweet fruits are balancing. Sour fruits are aggravating.

Vegetables: artichokes, asparagus, beets, broccoli, brussels sprouts, cauliflower, cucumbers, celery, green beans, Jerusalem artichokes, leafy greens, mushrooms, okra, parsley, peas, (sweet) potatoes, pumpkin, purslane, zucchini. Sweet and bitter vegetables are balancing.

Grains: basmati rice, millet, oats, quinoa; ancient wheat such as einkorn, emmer, or spelt

Legumes: All legumes are balancing, such as green, yellow, and red lentils; chickpeas, fava beans, kidney beans, mung beans, white beans, split peas, and tofu.

Dairy: butter (unsalted), ghee, mild fresh cheeses (mozzarella, ricotta, cottage cheese), cow or goat milk

Nuts and seeds: chia seeds, coconut, hempseeds, pumpkin seeds, sesame seeds, sunflower seeds

Oils: (unsalted) butter, coconut oil, ghee, olive oil (cold-pressed and unrefined)

Animal protein: eggs (especially egg whites), chicken and turkey (breast), (freshwater) or nonoily white fish

Sweeteners: coconut sugar, date syrup, maple syrup

Spices: coriander, cumin, dill, fennel, mint, saffron, turmeric

Drinks: coconut, oat, or rice milk; pomegranate or green juices; dandelion "coffee"; green or white tea; herbal teas (chamomile, dandelion, fennel, honeybush, jasmine, lemon balm, licorice, nettle, oat straw, peppermint, rose, rooibos); beer; dry white wine

## Regenerator (Kapha) or Late Winter and Spring Diet

Regenerators usually have a slow digestion, low appetite, and a tendency toward fullness, congestion, and excess weight. In late winter and spring (February until May), we can see a natural aggravation of Kapha dosha, with heaviness, congestion, mucous, and spring allergies. Since some of the qualities of Kapha are heavy, cold, and oily or moist, during spring we do best with foods that are light, dry, and warm, and the bitter, pungent, and astringent tastes.

### *Low-Carb and High-Veggie Diet*

In general, Regenerators do best with a low-carbohydrate diet, avoiding especially bread and pastries. Instead of grain-based carbohydrates like rice or bread, Regenerators do better getting the majority of their carbohydrate intake from vegetables, especially greens, artichokes, and cruciferous vegetables such as broccoli, cabbage, and cauliflower. Astringent fruits (berries, pomegranates) are more suitable than juicy fruits such as melons. Plant-based proteins (lentils, beans) are usually better suited than the heavier animal proteins. Especially cold and congestive dairy (milk, cheese, yogurt, ice cream) should be avoided, but a small amount of goat cheese or kefir with a generous sprinkling of black pepper can be an occasional treat.

#### Regenerator Foods

Balancing tastes: pungent, bitter, astringent
Balancing gunas: warm, light, dry
Fruit: apples, apricots, berries, cherries, pears, pomegranates. Sweet and sour fruits are aggravating. Astringent fruits are balancing.
Vegetables: artichokes, asparagus, beet greens, beets, broccoli, brussels sprouts, cabbage, carrots, cauliflower, eggplant, green beans, Jerusalem artichoke, leafy greens, leeks, mushrooms, okra, onions, parsley, peas, peppers, potatoes, purslane, spinach, sprouts, turnips. Pungent and bitter vegetables balance. Sweet, juicy vegetables aggravate.
Grains: basmati rice, buckwheat, corn (polenta), millet, rye

Legumes: All legumes are balancing such as red, yellow, and green lentils; black-eyed peas, chickpeas, fava beans, mung beans, navy beans, pinto beans, and split peas.

Dairy: Ghee. Avoid most other forms except small amounts of goat cheese and goat-milk kefir.

Nuts and seeds: chia seeds, flaxseeds, hempseeds, pumpkin seeds, sunflower seeds

Oil: ghee; coconut, hemp, olive, or flaxseed oils (unrefined and cold-pressed)

Animal products: eggs; chicken and turkey (breast); white-fleshed, nonoily fish (cod, sea bass, sea bream, snapper)

Sweeteners: honey

Spices: basil, black pepper, cardamom, chili, cinnamon, cloves, coriander, cumin, fenugreek, ginger, mint, mustard seeds, nutmeg, oregano, paprika, parsley, rosemary, sage, thyme, turmeric

Drinks: hemp or rice milk; pomegranate or green juices; white, green, or black tea; pu'erh tea; spicy chai; coffee; herbal teas (chamomile, cinnamon, clove, ginger, linden, nettle, rooibos, sage, thyme, tulsi); dry white or red wine

## It Is Not Just What You Eat: Combining Food for Optimal Digestion

While it is true that a person's agni largely determines how well a food is digested, food combinations are also of prime importance. When two or more foods having different tastes, energy, or digestive requirements are combined, agni can become overloaded. Poor food combinations can create fermentation and endotoxicity (*ama*) and lead to gas, bloating, indigestion, dysbiosis, and chronic inflammation. No wonder that today most over-the-counter medicines are digestive and dietary pills for stomach pain, acidity, bloating, and constipation.

### Top Four Reasons for Digestive Trouble

1. **Mismatch:** eating the wrong foods for our agni, constitution, or season

2. **Fast foods:** eating too much processed and fast foods (pizza, burgers, fries) or sugar (desserts, cookies, cakes)
3. **Untimely eating:** overeating, (emotional) eating when not hungry, or skipping meals despite being hungry
4. **Incompatible food combining:** eating foods with incompatible energetics and digestion times in the same meal

### *Think Twice About Eating That Smoothie Bowl*

Long-term poor food combining can cause doshic imbalance, toxicity, and disease. A classic example is combining yogurt, granola, and fruit, which most of us consider a "healthy" breakfast. This combo is incompatible because while fruit digests much faster than any other food (after all, it's just simple sugars), the yogurt is heavy, cold, and needs a much longer digestion time because of its fat and protein content. So the fruit sits fermenting in the digestive tract until the yogurt gets digested. This greatly diminishes agni, changes the intestinal flora, and produces ama, which leads to indigestion, dysbiosis, sinus congestion, allergies, cysts, and fibroids. The same applies to smoothie bowls, which often combine fresh fruits with heavy-to-digest nuts, seeds, and (plant-based) milk or yogurt.

### *Incompatible Food Combinations According to Ayurveda (Viruddha Ahara)*

| Don't Eat | With |
|---|---|
| Fruits | Anything |
| Milk | Anything (especially meals, fruits, fish, meat, yogurt, and cheese) |
| Meat/Fish | Dairy (milk, cheese, yogurt) |
| Yogurt | Fruit, meat, fish, eggs, dairy, hot drinks, nightshades |

If these rules feel a little overwhelming to you, I recommend starting with the two most important rules of food combining.

1. First, *eat fruit alone*, away from meals, and don't combine it, especially, with yogurt or milk.
2. Second, *do not eat dairy* (milk, cheese, yogurt) *with meat or fish*, such as meat with cream-based sauces or fish with yogurt dips such as tzatziki.

## Food Combining Upgrade from the Western Perspective

If somebody has weak agni and a lot of digestive trouble, in addition to the Ayurvedic food combining rules, I like to include a few key points from the Western nutritional perspective.

### *Rule 1: Place Highest-Protein Foods at the Beginning of the Meal*

The highest-protein foods have priority because they require greater amounts of stomach acid, whereas carbohydrates and other foods require very little. Foods with the highest amount of protein are animal products (meat, fish, dairy, eggs), legumes (beans, lentils), nuts, and seeds. When protein-rich foods are eaten after starches and other foods, the stomach acid will not be sufficient for their digestion. An example would be Spanish tapas or Turkish meze, where many different foods are eaten before the main protein course of fish or meat. Similarly, in Italy, eating pasta (carbohydrates) before the main protein-based (meat or fish) course. These are very difficult combinations.

### *Rule 2: Proteins, Fats, or Starches (Carbohydrates) Combine Best with Green and Non-Starchy Vegetables*

Greens and non-starchy vegetables (broccoli, cabbage, leek, spinach) are the foods best eaten at the same time with protein or starches. A concentrated protein (meat or fish) is also best digested if it is consumed in relatively small amounts. Fat and oils slow the digestion of protein, and thus a protein-rich meal should always be cooked with very little additional fat (butter, oil, or cream). People with compromised digestion do better with a single carbohydrate source per meal, such as one type of grain or starchy vegetables. For example, a burger with bun and fries is a very difficult combination because you are combining a protein with two heavy starches. A better idea would be to pair the burger patty or meatballs with a side salad or some steamed broccoli.

### *Rule 3: Fruit and Sweets Should Be Eaten Alone*

Because of their relatively simple carbohydrate structure, fresh fruits and concentrated sweeteners pose a special problem when combined with other foods. Since they digest much faster than anything else, they ferment, causing gas, bloating, and toxemia. Fruits and products made with sweeteners are best eaten by themselves at least two to three hours after or thirty minutes before a meal. The same applies to juices. In Ayurveda, we have a saying: "Always eat dessert first."

### *Simple Tricks to Offset Bad Food Combining*

Of course, there are factors that can lessen the effect of bad food combining, such as a strong digestive fire (*agni*), the use of spices and herbs, one-pot meals, and only indulging in bad combinations once in a blue moon.

- **Agni power:** A strong digestive fire is the most powerful tool of all to deal with "bad" food combinations, so keep your digestion strong and avoid overeating, eating cold and heavy foods, and eating leftovers.
- **Spice it up:** Spices and herbs are often used to make foods more compatible or to counteract difficult energetic effects—for example, by adding cinnamon to ice cream, cardamom to coffee, or cooling lassi (yogurt drink) to very spicy foods.
- **One-pot meals:** According to the Ayurvedic physician Dr. Robert Svoboda, if foods with different and possibly aggravating qualities—such as a mixture of vegetables, beans, grains, or meats—are cooked together in the same pot, "the various foods have settled their differences in the pot, fought out whatever needed to be fought out, and come to some conclusion, which you then consume."[5]
- **Don't repeat:** Finally, eating a bad combination occasionally is not detrimental. However, if something has become a daily

habit—such as yogurt and fruit daily for breakfast—it can lead to imbalance and serious health problems.

## Underrated Superfoods: The Power of Herbs and Spices

As we have seen, spices can be used not only to counteract the negative effects of certain foods but also for their potent medicinal properties—and, of course, for their amazing taste and flavor. Anybody who has traveled in India will remember the ample use of chili, mustard seeds, turmeric, and curry leaves in many of India's dal and sambar dishes; and many travelers to Southeast Asia cannot get enough of the fragrant curries cooked in coconut milk infused with ginger, turmeric, galangal, lime leaves, and lemongrass. Unfortunately, both in Europe and the United States, mainstream cuisine uses mostly salt and black pepper, and occasionally fresh herbs such as basil or thyme. This is such a shame given the rich historical use of spices for aromatic and medicinal purposes.

The following is an invitation to start your own personal medicinal and culinary spice cabinet. For me, spices are personalities, so I introduce them to you first very briefly—almost like speed dating—in groups that have similar personalities and actions. After, once your interest is piqued, you can read more about their individual superpowers, track records, and which dishes they like to hang out with.

### *The Personality Preview*

#### Belly Babes

This group of spices is fantastic for any kind of digestive trouble, especially indigestion, gas, and bloating.

Asafetida/hing: Our favorite digestive aid in Ayurveda, this sulfurous resin lends any dish a deliciously pungent and garlicky flavor.

Cinnamon: This all-rounder can be pulled out any time of the day—in your morning porridge, lunch soup, midafternoon apple pie, or dinner roast.

Cumin: This global star—slightly smoky and earthy, especially when roasted—is used in many Middle Eastern, Indian, and Mexican dishes. It goes exceptionally well with meat, beans, or lentils.

Fennel seed: Sweet and with a hint of licorice, fennel is excellent with meat or cabbage dishes. Simply roasted, it's a great breath freshener and digestive aid after meals.

Nutmeg: Way underused, this sweet and pungent nutlike spice is not only wonderful in baked goods but also fantastic in curries and pasta dishes. It pairs exceptionally well with sage and pumpkin.

### Fiery Flames

This spice gang excels at kick-starting a sluggish digestion and metabolism as well as remedying low appetite, mucous, congestion, and poor circulation.

Black pepper: Along with salt, black pepper is globally the most popular spice. It adds pungency and heat to any dish, as well as kick-starts your fat-burning metabolism.

Chili pepper: The boldest of all spices adds heat and kick to almost any dish and is a must in curries, Asian stir-fries, and Mexican dishes.

Cloves: A little goes a long way with this sweet and pungent spice. It is not only a star in the famous Indian masala chai tea but also a fantastic kitchen remedy for a toothache.

Ginger: Together with cinnamon. ginger is another all-rounder. It's fantastic in granola, wonderful in carrot soup, zesty in Asian stir-fries, and comforting as a warming winter tea.

### Soothing Squad

This group of spices is well-known for their ability to soothe acidity, heat, and inflammation.

Cardamom: An uplifting, exotic, aromatic Indian spice that is fantastic in coffee, desserts, and cookies.

Coriander: Used liberally in Indian, Asian, and Mexican cooking, coriander or cilantro is one spice that divides people. Some hate it and claim it tastes soapy, while others love its lemony bright flavor.

Saffron: The world's most expensive spice has a mild but distinct flavor and gives dishes a deep yellow color. It is used in desserts, teas, and most famously in international rice dishes such as Spanish paella, Italian risotto, and Iranian jeweled rice.

Turmeric: While its flavor is quite neutral, its color is gorgeously yellow. Turmeric is hands-down one of the most potent anti-inflammatory spices around, and a staple in curries and many rice dishes.

### Zesty Zing

This spice squad is known for its aromatic oils that help open lungs, uplift mood, support digestion, and increase circulation.

Bay leaf: This humble leaf has a stellar track record that goes back to ancient Greece. It adds a wonderfully earthy and bright flavor to soups, stews, fish, and pasta sauces.

Black cumin (nigella sativa): This traditional Middle Eastern powerhouse is a small black seed with a pungent and nutty flavor that adds depth and crunch to bread, Turkish flatbreads (*pide* or *börek)*, and pastries.

Rosemary: Lovely, strong pine-like taste that goes well with oven-baked potatoes and grilled meats, but also is unusually good sprinkled over summer-fruit tarts or in apricot jam.

Thyme: Another powerful and aromatic Mediterranean herb that can be used fresh or dried and is great with meat or roasted vegetables, as a spice rub, or infused into olive oil.

## The Spice Cabinet

### *Belly Babes*

**Asafetida/hing (*Ferula assafoetida*).** Our favorite digestive aid in Ayurveda, this sulfurous resin lends any dish a deliciously pungent and garlicky flavor.

Balances: Movers (Vata) and Regenerators (Kapha)
Aggravates: Transformers (Pitta)

Blackish brownish in color, this gum resin comes from the sap of a variety of giant fennel. It has a strong and slightly sharp odor and often comes crushed and mixed with rice flour into a powder that mitigates its intensity. Small amounts, however, give a beautiful onion-garlic flavor to dishes, especially in stews and curries. Asafetida is perhaps the most used digestive stimulant in Ayurveda, since it increases stomach fire and strengthens agni, removes gas and bloating from the intestines, destroys worms and pathogenic bacteria, and supports a healthy intestinal flora (fantastic for leaky gut and dysbiosis). On the mind, it acts like garlic, having a grounding effect. Due to its heating properties, asafetida increases Pitta, while reducing Vata and Kapha.

### * FUN FACTS

- While this spice is a staple in every curry, and many think it is quintessentially Indian, it is mostly imported from Afghanistan and Iran.
- The Persians used to call this spice "food of Gods," while the Romans were not so fond of it and aptly named it "smelly or fetid gum" (*asa foetida*).
- In Turkey, it is colloquially called "the back of the devil" (*şeytan-tersi*), mostly due to its sulfurous smell but also because it is still in some rural areas used for witchcraft and black magic. I remember when I first started buying large amounts of it at the spice bazaar in Eminönü, Istanbul, the sellers would eye me very suspiciously, probably thinking I was a foreign witch. Now they know what I do, and whenever I go there, we have a good laugh.

### HOW TO USE

- Since asafetida is a strong spice, a little goes a long way. A half teaspoon of the powder can be substituted for two minced garlic cloves or a half cup of minced onion. I always like to fry it in a little oil or ghee before I add other spices and vegetables.
- Because it is such a great carminative that prevents and settles gas and bloating, I always use it with beans or lentils and cruciferous vegetables such as cabbage or broccoli.

**Cinnamon (*Cinnamomum verum/zeylanicum/aromaticum*).** This allrounder can be pulled out any time of the day—in your morning porridge, lunch soup, midafternoon apple pie, or dinner roast.

Balances: Movers (Vata) and Regenerators (Kapha)
Aggravates: Transformers (Pitta)

Found in Indonesia, Sri Lanka, and Malaysia, cinnamon is an effective herb for strengthening digestion and harmonizing the flow of circulation. Cinnamon is a good diaphoretic and expectorant in colds and flu, especially for weak constitutions. Like ginger, cinnamon is almost a universal medicine, relieving muscle tension, strengthening the heart, and warming the kidneys. It is also used for loss of appetite, dyspepsia, intestinal spasms, gas, and bloating. Many studies have found cinnamon to be helpful in lowering blood glucose levels in type 2 diabetes as well as effectively reducing cholesterol. Warming, light, and dry in nature, cinnamon pacifies Vata and Kapha but can aggravate Pitta in excess. Keep in mind that not all cinnamon is the same. There are two distinctly different types: Ceylon cinnamon (*Cinnamomum verum/zeylanicum*) and cassia (*Cinnamomum aromaticum*). Cassia cinnamon is thicker and darker in color than its Ceylon counterpart, and because it is much cheaper, it makes up most of the cinnamon you see on supermarket shelves. Additionally, the cassia variety contains much more of the liver-damaging chemical coumarin, which can be problematic if you consume cinnamon in large amounts.

## ❊ FUN FACTS

- For all its worldwide and historical fame, Ceylon cinnamon is from the small island nation Sri Lanka, formerly known as Ceylon. The country still produces about 90 percent of the world's commercial Ceylon cinnamon.
- Ceylon cinnamon comes from the inner bark of a tree. The branches are cut off for harvesting and the bark peeled off. After peeling, the inner bark is rolled into quills, like a cigar, and hung up to dry before being sent to market.
- Cinnamon has been found to have insect-repelling properties and can be used in different forms, such as sprays, candles, or homemade bug repellent.

### HOW TO USE

- Use a cinnamon stick with fresh ginger as a lovely winter tea.
- Cinnamon is fantastic in your morning porridge or granola, cooked stewed apples, pear tarts, puddings, and cookies.
- I use it in many savory dishes, such as with a little cumin and nutmeg on oven-roasted carrots, in sweet potato soup, white bean stews, and lentil curries.
- If you sprinkle cinnamon on sliced apple or pear, it makes the fruits more Vata-friendly and less likely to cause gas or bloating.

**Fennel (*Foeniculum vulgare*).** Sweet and with a hint of licorice, fennel is excellent with meat or cabbage dishes. Simply roasted, it is a great breath freshener and digestive aid after meals.

Balances: Movers (Vata), Regenerators (Kapha), and Transformers (Pitta)

Fennel seeds are a flavorful and aromatic spice that have been used in cooking and traditional medicine for centuries. Sweet, pungent, and neutral, fennel balances all three doshas. It is one of the best herbs for digestion, strengthening agni without aggravating Pitta, stopping cramping, and dispelling flatulence. Mild yet effective, fennel seeds are excellent for digestive problems such as bloating or malabsorption, especially in children or the elderly. With a taste similar to that of anise, fennel seeds are a superb nervine, calming and relaxing while keeping the mind alert and focused. Fennel seeds promote menstruation and ease menstrual cramps. They also increase breast milk production in nursing mothers and are thus a vital part of many Ayurvedic postpartum herbal preparations. For urinary problems, they combine well with coriander seeds.

### ✻ FUN FACTS

- Fennel seeds are known for their ability to freshen breath and promote overall digestive health. In India, fennel seeds are mixed with other spices to create a colorful digestive known as *mukhwas*, which is found at the entrance of every restaurant and said to refreshen one's breath as well as support digestion.
- While India is the world's biggest manufacturer of fennel, the seeds are famously also part of the Chinese five-spice mixture, which includes star anise, cloves, cinnamon, and Szechwan peppercorns.

### HOW TO USE

- Use as a tea or with breads, crackers, and curries.
- I always dry-roast the seeds first, until their aroma is released and they turn golden. Then I grind the seeds with a mortar and pestle or a spice grinder and add them to meals or teas.
- Fennel goes exceptionally well with cabbage. Roast the seeds in ghee, add onions and thinly sliced white cabbage, and sauté until all caramelizes.

**Cumin (*Cuminum cyminum*).** Another global star. Slightly smoky and earthy, especially when roasted, cumin is used in many Middle Eastern, Indian, and Mexican dishes. It goes exceptionally well with meat, beans, or lentils.

Balances: Movers (Vata), Regenerators (Kapha), and Transformers (Pitta)
Aggravates: Transformers (Pitta) in excess

Cumin, like coriander, is an annual herb in the Apiaceae family. The cumin plant is native to Egypt and the Mediterranean region, and it is grown throughout the western Mediterranean, the Middle East, and parts of Asia. After black pepper, cumin is the second most popular spice in the world, first made popular by the Greeks and Romans. It has a warm, earthy aroma and flavor, with a hint of sweetness and bitterness. Cumin seeds are light, dry, and only slightly warm in nature. They subdue excess Vata and Kapha and can also be enjoyed in moderation by Pitta. They increase digestion and absorption, and are fantastic for gas, bloating, malabsorption, and diarrhea. Cumin seeds also have an affinity to the female reproductive system and are said to strengthen the uterus and remove impurities from the blood.

### ❋ FUN FACTS

- During the Middle Ages, cumin was believed to keep chickens and lovers from running away.
- Today, India is the largest producer and consumer of cumin seeds. It produces approximately 70 percent of the total cumin production in the world.

### HOW TO USE

- Whole cumin seeds are used at the beginning of the cooking process, dry-roasted or roasted in a little ghee to release their flavor.
- Even when a recipe calls for cumin powder, I first dry-roast the seeds and then freshly grind them into a powder. Try it and you will never go back to the ubiquitous powder.
- Use with pickles, lentils and beans, cruciferous vegetables such as broccoli or cabbage, and meat, and in Mexican or Indian dishes.

**Nutmeg (*Myristica fragrans*).** Way underused, this sweet and pungent, nutlike spice is not only wonderful in baked goods but also fantastic in curries and pasta dishes. Pairs exceptionally well with sage and pumpkin.

Balances: Movers (Vata) and Regenerators (Kapha)
Aggravates: Transformers (Pitta)

Native to the Moluccas or "Spice Islands" in the South Pacific, nutmeg is treasured for its unique flavor, nutty aroma, and medicinal properties. In Ayurveda, nutmeg is one of the most important Vata-reducing spices. It is useful in any kind of Vata-related disorder, particularly when there is nerve pain and cramping. Nutmeg is very useful for diarrhea and intestinal disorders, helps regulate agni, and increases the absorption of nutrients. Mixed with the Ayurvedic adaptogenic roots shatavari or ashwagandha, nutmeg is also considered a sexual stimulant or aphrodisiac. When used topically, nutmeg essential oil is helpful in relieving sore and inflamed joints and muscles. Large doses of nutmeg internally—more than five grams, or roughly one nut per day—can be hallucinogenic and toxic.

### ✻ FUN FACTS

- The fruit of the nutmeg tree, known as the nutmeg apple, resembles a peach in shape. When ripe, the fruit splits in half and reveals a small nut (nutmeg) that's embraced by a netting of red, waxy bands (mace). Mace, very similar to nutmeg in taste, is lesser known but also used as a slightly more peppery spice, especially in rice dishes.

### HOW TO USE

- Always buy the nut whole and grind it fresh since it has many valuable essential oils that evaporate quickly.
- A quarter nut grated and cooked into milk at night is a great insomnia remedy. Because its onset is delayed by at least three hours, either drink early or combine with a faster-acting herb such as poppy seed.
- Nutmeg is traditionally used in milk, cakes, and puddings, but I also like to use it in dal and pumpkin or lentil soup.

*Fiery Flames*

**Black Pepper (*Piper nigrum*).** Along with salt, black pepper is globally the most popular spice. It adds pungency and heat to any dish as well as kick-starts your fat-burning metabolism.

Balances: Movers (Vata) and Regenerators (Kapha)

Aggravates: Movers (Vata) long-term and in excess; Transformers (Pitta)

As a powerful digestive stimulant, black pepper is used in salads and heavier vegetable and meat dishes to help digestion. Dry, light, and pungent in nature, it helps conditions of excess mucous, as well as low appetite, indigestion, gas, and bloating. Black pepper is an excellent choice for cleansing ama (endotoxins) and excessive Kapha from the body. Due to its heating nature, it can increase Pitta and should be avoided in most inflammatory conditions. Due to its drying effect, long-term or excessive use can also increase Vata. Black pepper is a superb medicine for those suffering from coughs, cold, and asthma, especially when mixed with honey. Its active ingredient, piperine, has also been shown to boost metabolism and assist weight loss and fat reduction.

### ❋ FUN FACTS

- Black peppercorns are green when harvested and change color while drying. White peppercorns are black peppercorns without the skin. The most expensive red peppercorn variety occurs when the berries are left on the vine for longer than normal.
- Black pepper represents about 50 percent of a typical restaurant's spice usage.

### HOW TO USE

- Always grind black pepper freshly because when exposed to light and air, its pungent and potent active ingredient, piperine, transforms into the tasteless isochavicine. This is why the ground black pepper you see in most restaurants tastes like sawdust.
- Use with vegetable or meat dishes, beans, curries, and pasta.
- My teacher, Dr. Vasant Lad, always recommended that if you consume cheese—which is cold and mucous-producing—you should make sure to grind some black pepper over it to counteract its heavy and clogging nature.

**Chili Pepper (*Capsicum annuum*).** Chili, the boldest of all spices, adds heat and kick to almost any dish and is a must in curries, Asian stir-fries, and Mexican dishes.

Balances: Movers (Vata) and Regenerators (Kapha)
Aggravates: Movers (Vata) long-term and in excess; Transformers (Pitta)

All over the world, chili peppers have long been a favorite for spicing up hot dishes because of their pungent flavor. They are a great digestive, and they're antibacterial and antiparasitic. While considered a valuable medicine, chili peppers must be used with caution since overuse can strongly aggravate Pitta. Chili is a strong stimulant, both circulatory and digestive, and a powerful dispeller of internal cold. It can also serve as a diaphoretic in treating colds and flu. Effective for burning toxins and excess fat and stimulating digestion and metabolism, chili is a good choice for Kapha conditions involving cold, congestion, and obesity. Due to its *rajasic* (overstimulating) and drying qualities, however, excessive long-term use aggravates Vata, disturbs the mind, and causes excessive dryness and inflammation.

### ✻ FUN FACTS

- There are thousands of different types of chili peppers in the world.
- While Asian food without the heat of chili is unimaginable, chili is actually not native to India (or Southeast Asia, for that matter) but was introduced to the world from Central and South America only after the Spanish conquests of the 1500s.
- In the form of medicinal plasters and compresses, chili is often used externally for muscle spasms and painful arthritic joints.
- Some cultures put chili powder in their shoes to keep their feet warm.

### HOW TO USE

- Use chili in soups and curries; in Mexican, Indian, or Southeast Asian dishes; and as a condiment with a kick.
- When I travel in India or other hot countries where kitchen hygiene

may be an issue and food poisoning a possibility, I always order my dishes extra-spicy or with some chili on the side to kill any (possible) parasites or bacteria. This trick has never failed me.

**Cloves (*Syzygium aromaticum*).** With cloves, a little of this sweet and pungent spice goes a long way. It is not only a star in the famous Indian masala chai tea but also a fantastic kitchen remedy for toothache.

Balances: Movers (Vata) and Regenerators (Kapha)
Aggravates: Transformers (Pitta)

Cloves are the rich, brown, dried, unopened flower buds of *Syzygium aromaticum*, an evergreen tree in the myrtle family believed to be indigenous to the Moluccas, or Spice Islands, of Indonesia. They have a warm and pungent aroma while maintaining a strong, sweet flavor. With their very distinct and strong flavor, cloves are sprinkled onto chutneys, sauces, curry dishes, meat-based dishes, jam, and desserts. Cloves increase Pitta but pacify excess Kapha and Vata. They are astringent and an effective stimulant, appetizer, rejuvenator, and digestive aid. Cloves dispel cold, disinfect the lymph, and alleviate congestion. Out of all spices, cloves are highest in antioxidant capacity, in addition to being a powerful antibacterial, antiviral, and antifungal medicine. Cloves contain a very high amount of essential oils, including eugenol, which improves liver function, reduces inflammation, and decreases oxidative stress. In India, cloves are one signature ingredient in the famous Indian masala chai tea, along with ginger, cardamom, cinnamon, and black pepper.

### ✻ FUN FACTS

- The name *clove* is said to come from the French *clou*, meaning "nail," hinting at the unique shape of the clove buds.
- In ancient China, cloves were used as breath fresheners, and anybody having an audience with the emperor was obliged to chew some cloves.
- Today, oil of cloves is used as a painkiller for dental emergencies,

so if you have nothing else on hand, chew on a clove to relieve a toothache.

#### HOW TO USE

- Use in small amounts in Christmas cookies, spice cakes, and stewed fruit dishes.
- Cloves add a wonderful kick to chutneys and pickles.
- They pair well with onion, star anise, and peppercorns in savory bean or meat dishes.
- A traditional Chinese medicine remedy to support recovery of your lungs after a cold or bronchitis is half a pear, peeled and studded with eight to ten cloves and baked in the oven at 180°C for twenty to thirty minutes. After removing the cloves, you eat half a pear daily for at least one week.

**Ginger (*Zingiber officinale*).** Together with cinnamon, ginger is another all-rounder: fantastic in granola, wonderful in carrot soup, zesty in Asian stir-fries, and comforting as a warming winter tea.

Balances: Movers (Vata), Regenerators (Kapha), and Transformers (Pitta)
Aggravates: Transformers (Pitta) in dry form and/or in excess

Grown in China and India, ginger is a favorite spice of the tropical and subtropical regions. Just like turmeric, it is considered a universal medicine. The underground stem (known as the rhizome) of the ginger plant is what is used as a spice. So technically the ginger that we consume is not really a root but the rhizome. The flesh of the ginger rhizome can be yellow, white, or red in color, depending upon the variety. Fresh ginger is sweet, lightly pungent, and warming. In moderation, it balances all doshas, but—especially in dry form—it can aggravate Pitta and should be used with caution during summer. In fall and winter, however, ginger is a must-have for colds, cough, and congestion. Ginger juice, mixed with honey, relieves congestion in the lungs and facilitates breathing. Taken freshly grated with a squeeze of lemon, a pinch of salt and black pepper, and a few drops of honey before a meal, it kindles agni, increases secretion of digestive enzymes, and helps digestion. It also cures morning sickness, motion sickness, nausea, and vomiting. In general, ginger is a great warming and anti-inflammatory spice that enhances circulation, cures headaches and arthritis, and relieves gas and cramps in the abdomen (including menstrual cramps). It is also a great tonic for the heart.

### ✻ FUN FACTS

- The word *ginger* comes from the Sanskrit *srngavera* (*srnga*, "horn"; *vera,* "body"), most likely referring to the shape of ginger.
- As one of the first spices exported from the Orient, ginger arrived in Europe during the spice trade and was already used by ancient Greeks and Romans.
- Chinese medicine and Ayurvedic practitioners have relied on ginger for thousands of years for its anti-inflammatory properties and have used it as a superb catalyst, an herb that potentizes an herbal formula into being more effective in the body.
- In Japan, ginger is mostly used in the form of ginger pickles, called *gari* and *beni shoga,* where thin ginger slices are marinated either in sweet or umeboshi vinegar, often with the addition of red shiso (perilla) leaves, which gives them their characteristic pink color.

### HOW TO USE

- I use fresh ginger in almost everything, but it is particularly suited for curries, Asian stir-fries, teas, chutneys, and desserts.
- One of my favorite winter immune-boosting teas is fresh ginger cooked with a few Chinese red dates or goji berries.

*Soothing Squad*

**Cardamom (*Elettaria cardamomum*).** An uplifting, exotic, aromatic Indian spice that is fantastic in coffee, desserts, and cookies.

Balances: Movers (Vata), Regenerators (Kapha), and Transformers (Pitta)

Along with saffron and vanilla, cardamom is one of the world's most exotic spices, grown in the hills of southern India, Tanzania, Sri Lanka, and Guatemala. Cardamom belongs to the same botanical family as ginger and turmeric, the Zingiberaceae family. Cardamom seeds are sweet, pungent, fragrant, and aromatic and often used in desserts, baked goods, and drinks. Cardamom aids digestion and uplifts the mind and heart. Warm, light, and dry in nature, cardamom seeds are one of the safest digestive stimulants, awaking the spleen and pancreas and removing excess mucous from the stomach and lungs. Cardamom is close to neutral in temperature but in excess can slightly increase Pitta, while reducing Kapha and Vata. Cardamom seeds relieve nausea and morning sickness and stop vomiting.

### ✻ FUN FACTS

- According to Chinese folk wisdom, consuming cardamom tea is the secret to a long life.
- Added to milk or milk desserts such as rice pudding, cardamom counteracts milk's mucous-forming properties.
- Added to coffee, cardamom is said to help reduce coffee's acidity and buffer caffeine's stress on the adrenal glands. In the Middle East, it is a common practice to cook cardamom seeds with coffee.
- Chewing a few cardamom seeds works as a superb breath freshener, especially after spicy meals or dishes containing raw onion or garlic.

### HOW TO USE

- Because it very quickly loses flavor and potency, cardamom is best bought in the small green pods and ground fresh as needed.
- Cardamom is one of my favorite spices for cookies, cakes, and raw date balls.
- Kashmiri Kahwa tea is a wonderful blend of green tea, cardamom, clove, saffron, and rose.
- I also love to use cardamom in curries, pumpkin soup, and my morning porridge.

**Coriander (*Coriandrum sativum*).** Used liberally in Indian, Asian, and Mexican cooking, coriander or cilantro is one spice that divides people. Some hate it and claim it tastes soapy, while others love its lemony bright flavor.

Balances: Movers (Vata), Regenerators (Kapha), and Transformers (Pitta)

Coriander, also known as cilantro or Chinese parsley, is an annual herb in the Apiaceae family. It is native to the Middle East and southern Europe but is now cultivated throughout the world. Coriander is light, unctuous, and cooling. It balances all three doshas but is a prime choice for reducing Pitta and inflammation. Coriander seeds strengthen the urinary tract and are thus often used as a diuretic tea or cold infusion to cure urinary tract infections. Along with cumin and fennel, coriander seeds make a great tri-doshic digestive tea. Coriander leaf (cilantro) juice is effective for allergies, hay fever, and rashes, and the pulp can be applied externally for skin irritation.

### FUN FACTS

- Coriander's name comes from the Greek word *koris*, meaning a "stink bug." This is likely a reference to the strong aroma given off by the cilantro leaves when they are bruised.
- Most people perceive the taste of coriander leaves as tart and lemony, but about 10 percent of the population experience the taste of cilantro as soapy. This is linked to a gene that detects aldehyde chemicals, which also happens to be present in soap.

### HOW TO USE

- Fresh coriander leaves are an ingredient in many South Asian foods such as curries, chutneys, and salads; in Chinese and Thai dishes; and in Mexican cooking, particularly in salsa and guacamole.
- As heat diminishes their flavor, coriander leaves are often used raw or added to the dish immediately before serving.
- Together with mint, ginger, and roasted coconut, fresh coriander leaves make a mean chutney.
- Like garlic, chlorella, and barlauch, coriander leaves are also shown to

bind to mercury, so I always make sure to eat some when I have fish or seafood.

**Saffron (*Crocus sativus*).** Saffron has a mild but distinct flavor and gives dishes a deep yellow color. It is used in desserts, teas, and most famously in international rice dishes such as Spanish paella, Italian risotto, and Iranian jeweled rice.

Balances: Movers (Vata), Regenerators (Kapha), and Transformers (Pitta)

Saffron is a spice derived from the flower of the *Crocus sativus* plant, also known as the "saffron crocus." It is often called "red gold" because it is the most expensive spice in the world. No wonder, because seventy-five thousand crocus flowers are required to prepare one pound of saffron threads or stigmas, all hand-harvested one by one. Saffron's name roots down to the Arabic word *zafran*, meaning "yellow," as a few strands render a beautiful yellow color to any rice dish or dessert. From an Ayurvedic point of view, saffron is light, subtly warming, and slightly bitter in taste. While saffron is considered tri-doshic, it is especially beneficial for balancing Vata and Kapha, while also gently pacifying excess Pitta when used in small amounts. Saffron is an important tonic for the female reproductive system. It has a specific affinity to the blood (*rakta dhatu*), and through this also nourishes the uterus, which is why it is usually recommended in cases of infertility. Saffron is also often used together with arjuna as a heart tonic or combined with turmeric or bhumyamalaki as a liver tonic. In addition to being investigated as a potent anticarcinogen,[6] it is also one of the most potent herbal catalysts in formula-making since it affects all tissues in the body and increases the potency of any herb it is mixed with.

## ✻ FUN FACTS

- Alexander the Great made use of Persian saffron as a cure for combat wounds during his Asia expeditions.
- Before seeing a male suitor, Cleopatra would bathe in saffron-infused milk.

- Today, Iran dominates the global production of saffron, accounting for about 90 percent of the yearly harvest.
- Fake saffron is often made from look-alikes such as safflower, turmeric, and dyed corn silk. You can spot fake saffron by performing a simple water test. When you add a few threads to a glass of water, genuine saffron will slowly release its color, turning the water a vibrant yellow color while the threads remain red. Fake saffron will either release the color too quickly or not at all, and the threads may lose their color completely.

**HOW TO USE**

- The deep red color signifies how good the saffron is because it signifies a higher concentration of crocin, its active ingredient that is responsible for its deep red color.
- It takes around ten to fifteen minutes of soaking for authentic saffron to change the color of the water. The thin strands of saffron will continue to infuse flavors for up to twelve hours when mixed with hot liquid.
- Kashmiri Kahwa tea is a wonderful blend of green tea, cardamom, clove, saffron, and rose.
- Saffron is beautiful when added to rice dishes or desserts, or infused into milk.

**Turmeric (*Curcuma longa*).** Its flavor is quite neutral, but turmeric's color is gorgeously yellow. It is hands-down one of the most potent anti-inflammatory spices around, and a staple in curries and many rice dishes.

Balances: Movers (Vata), Regenerators (Kapha), and Transformers (Pitta)
Aggravates: Movers (Vata) and Transformers (Pitta) long-term and in excess

Turmeric is easily one of the most powerful medicines in our spice cabinet. Its active ingredient, the polyphenol curcumin, is one of the most widely researched compounds in medical literature today. Bitter and astringent in taste and slightly heating in thermal nature, it balances Kapha dosha especially but can also be enjoyed by Vata and Pitta constitutions in moderation. It is the only spice that purifies, builds, and moves blood, making it important for many menstrual problems such as PMS, fibroids, cysts, or irregular cycles. Turmeric is a great source of beta-carotene. It strengthens digestion, kills worms, subdues excess gas and bloating, and helps improve intestinal flora. It is an excellent natural antibiotic and a superb anti-inflammatory and pain reliever, making it a great adjunct for inflammatory conditions such as heart disease, rheumatoid arthritis, and inflammatory bowel conditions such as colitis or diverticulitis. Turmeric cures skin diseases due to blood toxicity, such as eczema, psoriasis, and acne; and it helps to regulate blood sugar in diabetics. New medical research also reveals curcumin's anticancer potency.[7] Adding black pepper to turmeric in cooking or to an herbal formula potentiates the bioavailability of curcumin, an important antioxidant, anti-arthritic, and anticancer constituent.

### ✻ FUN FACTS

- Turmeric originates in southern India and Indonesia, and has a long history of use as a spice and medicine.
- Aside from its "superstar" active ingredient, curcumin, turmeric contains more than three hundred naturally occurring components including beta-carotene, ascorbic acid, calcium, flavonoids, fiber, iron, niacin, potassium, and zinc.
- Turmeric is also said to cleanse the chakras and subtle channels (*nadis*) of the body. It is often used in Hindu religious ceremonies and rituals.

### HOW TO USE

- I use turmeric in *everything*! It's particularly good in vegetable dishes, soups, curries, and rice.
- Keep in mind that curcumin, the main active ingredient in turmeric, is fat-soluble, which means it needs to be eaten with oil (and a pinch of black pepper) to aid absorption.
- A superb nutritional medicinal preparation is medicated Turmeric

Ghee (see page 235). It can be used daily as a substitute for butter on bread, as well as in baking and cooking.

- Golden milk (boiling milk with turmeric and ginger) is a classic Ayurvedic remedy for restful sleep, as an anti-inflammatory, and for strong immunity.
- For cold and cough, mix equal parts turmeric and honey with a little black pepper and lick a spoonful of it every few hours.

### *Zesty Zing*

**Bay Leaves (*Laurus nobilis*).** The humble bay leaf has a stellar track record that goes back to ancient Greece. It adds a wonderfully earthy and bright flavor to soups, stews, fish, and pasta sauces.

Balances: Movers (Vata) and Regenerators (Kapha)
Aggravates: Transformers (Pitta)

Bay leaves are a standard European cooking ingredient in many savory dishes such as soups, stews, and sauces. Though available fresh, typically they are easier to find dried. Bay leaves are part of the evergreen bay laurel family, native to the Mediterranean. The two most common types are Turkish, with long oval leaves; and Californian, with long narrow leaves. Slightly pungent and highly aromatic, bay leaves are a cardiovascular tonic, and they stimulate appetite and promote digestion. Hot and dry in nature, they reduce Vata and Kapha, thus they are particularly beneficial when used in foods that are considered mucous-producing. (The essential oil is fantastic for opening lungs and sinuses.) Bay leaves also help reduce gas and bloating and are thus often cooked with gas-producing foods such as lentils and beans. Indian bay leaf, *tamalpatra* (*Cinnamomum tamala*), is a slightly different species but is also often used in Ayurveda as a tea for colds, bloating, and indigestion.

## ✻ FUN FACTS

- Historically, the medicinal use of bay leaf was always important. Along with garlic, it was used to protect against epidemics and as an antirheumatic. It was drunk as a tea and used in baths, and the Romans used both leaves and berries for the treatment of liver disorders.

- There is a rich mythological history of use of bay leaves in ancient Greece, where it was the herb of poets, warriors, statesmen, and doctors. Famously, its leaves were made into wreaths to crown heroes and victorious athletes.

#### HOW TO USE

- Use bay leaves in soups, lentil or bean dishes, and pasta sauces. I almost always throw in one or two bay leaves with any lentil or bean dish I cook, as well as in bone broth, for better digestibility.
- In a classical Indian pilau rice, bay leaves combine gorgeously with black pepper, cinnamon, cardamom, and cloves.

**Black Cumin (*Nigella sativa*).** Black cumin, a traditional Middle Eastern powerhouse, is a small black seed with a pungent and nutty flavor that adds depth and crunch to bread, Turkish flatbreads (*pide* or *börek*), and pastries.

Balances: Movers (Vata) and Regenerators (Kapha)
Aggravates: Transformers (Pitta)

Reportedly found in Tutankhamun's tomb, black cumin is famous as an ancient sacred spice and medicine. Black cumin has a pungent, bitter, and smoky taste, and its seed is a beautiful and unusually black color. According to the famous Arabic physician Ibn Sina (Avicenna)'s *Canon of Medicine*, black cumin restores the body's energy and helps recovery from fatigue and low spirits. For centuries, black cumin has been used extensively in Unani (Islamic) medicine for asthma, bronchitis, coughs, rheumatism, and other inflammatory diseases. From an Ayurvedic perspective, black cumin is strengthening and helps build agni. It is also used to treat eczema and other skin conditions. In Chinese medicine, like other black foods (black beans, black sesame, black rice), black cumin is a strong kidney tonic. It can help reduce the size of kidney stones and strengthen overall kidney function. Black cumin is an immunomodulator, and its antitumor effects are beneficial for cysts and tumors of the abdomen, pancreas, and liver. Today, black cumin oil is widely popular and used internally for allergies, inflammatory conditions, and many forms of cancer.

### ✻ FUN FACTS

- The *Tibb-e-Nabawi* (medicine book of the Prophet Muhammad) reports that the only disease black cumin cannot cure is death. Its many uses have earned it the nickname "seed of blessing."
- Nearly all names of *Nigella sativa* in various cultures contain some form of the word *black*. In India, black cumin is called *kala jeera.*

### HOW TO USE

- Traditionally used in the Middle East on bread and pastries, I like to use the seeds sprinkled on salads or on top of vegetables, meat dishes, or curries.
- Due to their pungent and heating properties, which stimulate *agni* (digestive fire), black cumin seeds help break down mucous-increasing foods like yogurt or cheese.
- A traditional Chinese remedy for low energy and adrenal depletion is to mix a half teaspoon of black cumin seeds with honey and take this on an empty stomach in the morning, especially during the fall and winter seasons or during times of stress.

**Rosemary (*Rosmarinus officinalis*).** Rosemary's lovely, strong, and pine-like taste goes well with oven-baked potatoes and grilled meats, but it is also unusually good sprinkled over summer fruit tarts or in apricot jam.

Balances: Movers (Vata) and Regenerators (Kapha)
Aggravates: Transformers (Pitta)

Rosemary has a long history of both culinary and medicinal use. It is a perennial evergreen that grows in bushes with wood-like stems and short, pine-like needles. Rosemary is often grown as an ornamental shrub because it is extremely sturdy. Along with sage and mint, rosemary is a member of the botanical family Lamiaceae.

Rosemary's genus name, *Rosmarinus*, is from the Latin *ros* (dew) and *marinus* (sea). Growing in arid Mediterranean conditions, it survives on the mere humidity carried by the sea breeze, as its name implies. Aromatic, pungent, and slightly bitter, rosemary is a warming diaphoretic and digestive and, as such, is used for many Vata- and Kapha-related ailments. It stimulates the central nervous system, making it useful in cases of low blood pressure, fatigue, and sluggishness. As a circulatory stimulant, it is traditionally used to improve memory as well as to help with hair loss and dandruff. Taken internally as a tea or used externally as an oil in massage oils and rubs, rosemary combats muscle fatigue as well as pain and inflammation. Rosemary also has an affinity to the heart and circulation, and can mitigate oxidative damage, circulation issues, and irregular heartbeats, and generally strengthen the heart and circulation.

## FUN FACTS

- In ancient Greece, rosemary was used to fumigate temples and as an herb for garlands worn on the heads of scholars to improve memory and invigorate the spirit.
- Rosemary was associated with Athena, the goddess of wisdom, poetry, and arts.
- In ancient Rome, rosemary was a universal symbol of remembrance and used at funerals.

### HOW TO USE

- You can use rosemary in dried and fresh forms. Its piney, peppery, lemony, and woodsy flavor pairs well with most dishes, but pairs exceptionally well with bread (rosemary focaccia), oven-roasted potatoes, white bean stews, and lentil soups.
- As a highly aromatic herb that contains volatile oils that stimulate digestive enzymes and bile flow, rosemary is also often paired with harder-to-digest animal protein such as meat, chicken, or fish.

- I like to add a sprig of fresh rosemary with the stem intact to soups and stews and then remove it prior to serving.
- Often I submerge a sprig of rosemary, one or two cloves of garlic, and (organic!) lemon rind into a bottle of olive oil and use this beautifully aromatic oil drizzled over salads or vegetable dishes.

**Thyme (*Thymus vulgaris*).** Thyme is another powerful and aromatic Mediterranean herb that can be used fresh or dried and is great with meat or roasted vegetables, as a spice rub, and infused into olive oil.

Balances: Movers (Vata) and Regenerators (Kapha)
Aggravates: Transformers (Pitta)

Thyme is an aromatic and pungent herb of the mint family (Lamiaceae) known for the peppery aroma and flavor of its dried leaves and buds. Thyme is native to the Mediterranean and is cultivated throughout the world. From an Ayurvedic point of view, thyme is pungent and sharp, slightly bitter and drying, making it an excellent remedy for cold, cough, and congestion, as well as digestive trouble such as bloating and indigestion. Due to its antifungal and antibacterial properties, thyme is often used alongside garlic for fungal and bacterial infections. It balances Vata and Kapha but can be Pitta provoking, especially if used in excess.

### ✻ FUN FACTS

- Ancient Greeks strongly believed in the power of thyme and used it in battle to restore physical strength and vitality, promote bravery, and revive the spirit.
- Thyme was also used as an incense for ritual altar fires.

### HOW TO USE

- As with bay leaf, thyme is slow to release its flavor, so it is usually added early in the cooking process.
- Thyme is a basic ingredient in many Mediterranean and Middle Eastern cuisines. In France, it is one of the ingredients in the spice mix

herbes de Provence, and in bouquet garni, a bundle of herbs wrapped in a cheesecloth that is added to the pot while cooking and removed before serving.

- In Turkey, thyme tea (*zahter çayı*) is used as a digestive after meals.
- My favorite use of thyme is in the aromatic Middle Eastern blend za'atar, which also contains toasted sesame seeds, sumac, and salt. In Levantine countries, za'atar is often eaten by dipping a piece of flatbread into olive oil and then the spice mixture. However, it also goes exceptionally well sprinkled over salads, roasted vegetables, and soups.

### *Churnas—Spice Blends*

In cooking, spices generally appear in familiar blends and combinations. From garam masala in India, to za'atar in Lebanon and dukkah in Egypt, kitchens around the world employ traditional spices to give flavor and zest to their meals. In Ayurvedic cooking, we call these spice combinations *churnas* (which literally means "powder" in Sanskrit). We use churnas in Ayurvedic cooking for flavor as well as their superb medicinal and digestive effects. To enliven a churna's potency or healing property, it can be sautéed in a little ghee or olive oil for a minute, then drizzled over steamed vegetables, bean dishes, soups, or rice. I love making different mixtures from around the world and have them ready in my kitchen. They help transform even the simplest meal into an exotic adventure. Here are some of my favorites:

#### Africa

*Dukkah:* An Egyptian mix of toasted nuts and seeds such as hazelnuts, sesame seeds, coriander, and cumin.

*Harissa*: A fiery red paste made from smoked peppers and widely featured in Tunisian and other North African cuisines.

*Ras el hanout:* A varying blend of over twenty-five spices used in Moroccan cooking. It includes cinnamon, cardamom, rose, paprika, and cumin.

### Asia

*Chinese five spice:* A little of this pungent mix goes a long way, giving dishes a balanced hit of sweet, savory, and bitter. It includes star anise, Szechuan pepper, clove, cinnamon, and fennel seeds.

*Gomasio:* A Japanese condiment of toasted sesame seeds ground up with coarse sea salt. Especially delicious over rice.

### India

*Curry:* An Indian-inspired British invention, this popular mix typically includes turmeric, coriander, cumin, fenugreek, and chili.

*Garam masala: Garam* means "warm" or "hot," and the mix usually contains warming spices like cinnamon and cardamom.

### Middle East

*Advieh:* A Persian mix of dried rose petals and spices such as cinnamon, cardamom, cloves, nutmeg, and cumin. Often used in rice and stews.

*Za'atar:* A fragrant and tangy blend of thyme, sesame seeds, salt, and sumac.

If you want to experiment with making your own churna for your unique digestive needs and taste, you can choose from the list below:

Mover (Vata) digestion: irregular appetite, constipation, bloating
Spices: asafetida/hing, bay leaf, black cumin, cardamom, cinnamon, cumin, fennel, ginger, rosemary, saffron

Transformer (Pitta) digestion: hyperacidity, indigestion, loose stools
Spices: cardamom, coriander, cumin, fennel, saffron, turmeric

Regenerator (Kapha) digestion: lack of appetite, slow digestion
Spices: asafetida/hing, bay leaf, black pepper, black cumin, cardamom, chili, cinnamon, clove, coriander, ginger, rosemary, saffron, thyme, turmeric

Two famous Ayurvedic formulas that are widely used for all kinds of digestive troubles are briefly explained below. The detailed recipes are in the recipe section of the book:

Trikatu Churna (Fire Up Spice): Translated as "the three pungents"—dried ginger, black pepper, and Indian long pepper (*pippali*)—this blend is a fantastic kick for Regenerators as well as everybody with sluggish digestion, congestion, cold, allergies, or excess weight. I like to call this formula Fire Up Spice because of its immediate effect to kick-start agni strongly.

Hingvasthak Churna (Tame the Flame Spice): Translated as "hing plus eight," this mix has hing (asafetida) as its main star, featured alongside eight other digestive spices including cumin, ajwain, ginger, and black pepper. It is one of the best spice mixtures for weak and irregular digestion with gas, bloating, and malabsorption. I refer to this mix often as Tame the Flame Spice because of its unique ability to regulate digestion and absorption.

# 6

## Hack 3: Regenerate

### Dial Yourself into Longevity and Antiaging

The bamboo that bends is stronger than the oak that resists.
—Japanese proverb

### Why Physical and Mental Resilience Is Vital: An Ayurvedic and Western Medicine Perspective

Having stressors is part of human life, and, in fact, not all stress is bad. Our mind and body need challenges—just think of your cold morning shower, the pressure of weights in strength training, or the productivity benefit of a deadline. Stressors serve as opportunities to stimulate self-healing mechanisms and increase growth potential. The term *stress* emerged out of the field of engineering, where it was used to describe the actual physical strain put on a structure. By itself, a strain is not necessarily something negative. However, if there is too much weight or pressure exerted on the structure, it collapses. Similarly, in our body, if the stressors are prolonged and outweigh our skills and resources—be it poor diet, chronic illness, difficult relationships, or overworking—they start disrupting nearly every system in our body. Chronic stress suppresses the immune system, upsets our digestive and reproductive functions, increases inflammation and risk of cardiovascular disease, and accelerates aging.

### Be as Resilient as Bamboo

Throughout Asia, the bamboo tree is a popular symbol of uprightness and resiliency, and is used as a strong and flexible building material. When storms or heavy winter snow weigh on the bamboo tree, it is forced to bend almost to the ground. Yet when the storm subsides or the snow melts, the bamboo immediately snaps back to its full height. This is the embodiment of resilience: the ability to adjust to or recover easily from change, challenge, and adversity.

## Clean Lymph and Calm Mind = High Resiliency

From the Ayurvedic perspective, how physically and mentally resilient you are depends largely on two main buffer systems: your lymphatic tissue (*rasa dhatu*) and your nervous system (*majja dhatu*). When our body is properly nourished, our lymphatic system clean and responsive, and our mind calm and feeling safe, then our internal environment is tuned in to regeneration. It can easily adapt to and accommodate changes or stressors in the external environment. As a result, we recover faster. However, when our lymphatic system is stagnant, toxic, or depleted and our nervous system frazzled, it is much harder to deal with stressors of any kind.

Fortunately Ayurveda excels at providing us with many tools and practices to cultivate resilience. We have already covered how you can optimize your ability to *flow* and *transform* through recalibrating your circadian wiring and strengthening your digestive and metabolic power. Now we are ready to go one step further: You ignite your potential to *regenerate* through optimizing lymphatic flow and fortifying your nervous system.

## How to Regenerate

### *Rasa: Why Your Lymph Tissue May Be the Crucial Factor for Health and Physical Resilience*

The lymphatic tissue (*rasa dhatu*) is one of the seven basic tissues, or dhatus (*dhatu*, "that which holds"), that make up the human body and are fundamental to health because they make up who we are and provide both nourishment and support.[1] Rasa is so crucial because, as the first tissue to be formed after we ingest food, it is the precursor to all the other tissues. Like a river embodying all the different "waters," rasa circulates through the body, nourishing other tissues and organs and flushing out wastes. From a Western point of view, these internal waters are our plasma or the noncellular portion of the blood, which includes lymph and interstitial fluids. Closely related to Kapha dosha—both share similar qualities such as cool, moist, smooth, fluid, and cloudy—rasa is responsible for nourishment, immunity, and regeneration of the body.

### *Rasa = Juice = Nourishment*

*Rasa* is a Sanskrit word with multiple meanings. One of them is "juice" or "essence." ("Mercury" and "semen" are among the others.) In the previous chapter, we encountered rasa as the taste of food (*shad rasa*, "the six tastes"), which is experienced by the physical body, most notably on the taste buds of your tongue. In addition to the six tastes perceived on the tongue, there are also the nine tastes of emotions (*nava rasa*), which are experienced by the mind (*manas*).[2] So rasa dhatu is built through not only the taste (rasa) of our food but also the flavor of our emotions.[3] Together they affect and shape our primary tissue, rasa dhatu, "the mother of all tissues."

### *Rasa Is Both Nourishment and Waste Management*

Rasa is so vital for our health because, aside from nourishing the body and organs, it helps to clear cellular and metabolic wastes. Essentially it is like a gigantic garbage truck that collects waste from our organs and cells, funnels it into the lymphatic channels, and finally moves it out via lymph nodes into our kidneys and liver. According to Ayurveda, as the first tissue formed after digestion, rasa is very closely related to our digestive health and strength (*agni*). Western science supports this connection: two-thirds of our immune system is literally located in our digestive tract in the form of actual lymph (GALT, or gut-associated lymphoid tissue) and gut bacteria that communicate with it. How well we digest, absorb, assimilate, and eliminate food makes or breaks our physical resilience and immunity.

### *Are You Juicy, Dried Up, or Stagnant?*

When rasa is excellent (*rasa sara*), our skin is soft, smooth, and shining. We feel juicy, look juicy, and—most importantly—have the juice and power to act as needed. Our mind is clear and calm, our stamina good, and our immune system strong. When rasa dhatu is depleted (*rasa kshaya*)—often due to malabsorption, poor diet and lifestyle, or stress—it shows as dehydration, dry skin and mucous membranes, exhaustion, fatigue, absent menstruation, hypersensitivity (especially to sounds), and feeling easily overwhelmed. In this case, *rasayana*, or "rejuvenating therapies," are called for.

### *Most of Us Are Clogged Up*

For most people today—due to sedentary lives, stress, and a diet heavy in sugar, poor-quality animal protein, and processed foods—rasa dhatu is stagnant and congested (*rasa vrddhi*). Just as a river that is stagnant and does not flow can become filled with debris, toxins, and bacteria, stagnant lymph can become filled with cellular waste, toxins, and other substances that can impair immune function and create an environment that is conducive to inflammation and disease. Symptoms of stagnant or congested rasa are puffy eyes, water retention, lethargy, heaviness, nausea, high blood sugar and cholesterol, and lymphatic swelling or tender lymph nodes. Untreated, stagnant lymph can—along with chronic inflammation and toxicity—be a major contributing factor to chronic and autoimmune diseases, including cancer.

### *The Best Way to De-Stagnate Lymph Is Fasting*

When rasa dhatu is stagnant and congested, or when there is too much toxicity (*ama*) in the system, fasting is the best remedy. Fasting can be as simple as skipping a meal when you are not hungry, practicing twelve to sixteen hours of intermittent fasting (IF), doing a short reset cleanse, or initiating a longer (seasonal) detox. Fasting activates your garbage collectors—the specialized cells that scavenge for and eliminate oxidative damage, pathogens, and damaged and (pre)cancerous cells. Fasting is also an inexpensive (!) and highly effective way to reduce inflammation and reverse dysbiosis. Your cells become smarter, your mind sharper, and your body less prone to disease. In the following section, we will look at four effective ways of incorporating fasting into your daily life. If you have never done a fast, I recommend trying step 1 first and then slowly working your way into the longer fasts.

## Four Ways of Fasting That Activate Cell Autophagy and Repair

### *1. Skip: Avoid Snacking and/or Skip Meals*

One of the simplest ways to give your system a chance to deal with stagnant lymph or excess ama is to simply avoid snacking and only eat when you get a strong sign that you are actually hungry. Most of us eat out of habit or when food is put in front of us, no matter whether our digestive system is ready or not. Additionally, frequent snacking, overeating, eating too late, or emotional eating disrupts cellular metabolism. If you overeat or eat late at night, you can make it a habit to skip breakfast the next day and sip on hot water or ginger tea until a clear sign of hunger develops.

### *2. Give a Break: Intermittent Fasting (IF)*

I already briefly talked about the Ayurvedic view on intermittent fasting (IF), a pattern of time-restricted eating where you cycle between periods of eating and periods of fasting. There are different ways to practice intermittent fasting, but the most common methods involve limiting your calorie intake during certain hours of the day or days of the week. For example, the 16/8 method involves restricting eating to an eight-hour window each day and fasting for the remaining sixteen hours. The 5/2 method involves eating normally for five days of the week and restricting calorie intake to between five hundred and six hundred calories for two nonconsecutive days.

While both yoga and Ayurveda were using fasting (*upavasa*) spiritually and therapeutically long before IF became a popular practice, IF is now widely studied for many potential health benefits, such as improving insulin sensitivity, reducing inflammation, and promoting cellular repair. The type of intermittent fasting should always be tailored to your constitution and imbalance. In my experience, IF works best after a few weeks of lifestyle and nutritional optimization, such as in our nine- or eighteen-week Ayurveda 2.0 journey.

### *3. Mini Fasts: Personalized Short Fasts*

Practicing short mini fasts (24–48 hours) is a useful way to reset digestion and metabolism, especially after a period of overeating, a lot of eating out, or eating processed and fast foods. My teacher, Dr. Vasant Lad, suggests you determine which day of the week you were born, and then on that day every week (or once a month), you fast as a way of honoring your birth. This is a wonderful way of resetting your digestion and can be done according to your metabolic body type.

- Regenerators do best fasting on plain hot water, (mild) ginger tea, or vegetable broth.
- Transformers excel on a fast with water and (green) vegetable juices.
- Movers do best with a mono-diet fast of warm soups, Chinese congee, or Ayurvedic kitchari.

It is best to prepare the body for one to two days prior to the fast by slowly reducing taxing foods and drinks (alcohol, coffee, dairy, gluten, sugar, meat), strengthening agni (through spices), and priming the organs and channels for elimination (hydrotherapy as well as liver- and kidney-supportive teas).

### *4. Seasonal Reset: Longer Cleanses*

Throughout the year, the elements and doshas change (accumulate, peak, and wane) in the body. This is considered a natural process—for example, in winter, we accumulate excess Kapha (water and earth elements) or yin (building, nourishing, moistening) qualities in the form of a few more pounds or extra belly fat. In summer, we naturally accumulate Pitta (fire element) or yang (heating, energizing, lightening) qualities, which can express as excess body heat, rashes, and dryness. Detoxifying or fasting seasonally, from this point of view, is a way of resetting the body's balance and natural ability to heal itself. It helps get rid of toxins, doshas, and wastes accumulated in the previous season (doshas and ama) and prepare for optimal health in the coming season.

**Optimal Seasons for Detoxification: Spring and Fall.** Winter is the time of extreme yin. It is a time to move inward, hibernate, rest, nourish, and (re)build. Summer is the time of extreme yang. During this time, our energy is moving outward; it disperses and the digestive fire (*agni*) is weakened. In winter, we do not fast or detoxify because the body will not let go of toxins; it is naturally programmed to hold on to and store fat. This is why winter is also not a good time for dieting or focusing on weight loss goals. Our biorhythm is not programmed to shed excess weight in winter because evolutionarily it needed fat for insulation and energy. In summer, our energy and digestive power are already weakened and dispersed by the heat, so this is also not a good time to detoxify or undergo a strict fasting program, since the body already is depleted. Rather, according to Ayurveda and Chinese medicine, it is at the transformational juncture of the seasons (*sandhi*), in fall and spring, that we prepare for the coming season through a gentle cleanse or fast.

## How to Do a Spring Reset

Spring, according to Ayurveda, is the season of Kapha dosha and the earth and water elements. In Chinese medicine, it is the season of the wood element, which rules the liver and gallbladder. It follows a heavy winter diet rich in protein and fat, which has led to an accumulation of excess yin and Kapha dosha, needed in winter for insulation and energy. But just as the snow melts in the mountains, so in spring Kapha (mucous) melts in the body and can lead to spring allergies, congestion, heaviness, and stagnation. Thus in spring we focus on lightening the load on our overwhelmed digestive system as well as the most important detoxifying organ, the liver. Spring is an ideal time to clear away toxins and accumulations and make way for new growth in life—more energy, focus, and creativity.

### *Elimination Diet and Juice Fasting for Your Liver*

A gentle yet highly effective cleanse during spring is an elimination diet followed by a one- or two-day juice fast. For about one week, eliminate taxing foods and drinks from your diet: alcohol, sugar, coffee, animal products, gluten, and all processed foods. Focus on eating mostly plants, with plenty of fresh vegetables and fruits, accompanied by beans and lentils and alkalinizing whole grains such as millet and basmati rice. In addition, drink plenty of water and herbal teas such as chamomile, ginger, mint, lemon balm, or nettle. If you have experience with fasting and have no problems with blood sugar irregularities, you can follow this week of elimination diet with an additional day or two of juice fasting. This is a fantastic way of cleansing the liver and gallbladder, shedding excess pounds, and improving energy and metabolism.

## How to Do a Fall Reset

Fall is the season of Vata dosha and the ether and air elements. In Chinese medicine, it is the season of the metal element, which rules the lungs and the large intestine. Just as the leaves lose color and start drying up and October winds bring cooler temperatures, so do our bodies make a transition into winter mode. The focus of a fall cleanse is to clear away the accumulated summer heat, optimize the immune system, and lubricate the body for winter. We use external oil (massage) and internal oleation (drinking ghee) to nourish deep tissues and pull fat-soluble toxins from the tissues and purge them.

### *Fall Is Perfect for a Mini Panchakarma*

A gentle yet highly effective cleanse during fall is a mini version of panchakarma, the traditional Ayurvedic cleansing program. It is wonderfully soothing to the digestive and nervous systems. During the preparation phase, which is at least four days but ideally one week, you avoid all taxing foods and drinks—alcohol, coffee, sugar, animal products, gluten, and all processed foods. You focus on eating freshly cooked vegetables, fruits, beans or lentils, eggs, nuts, and wholesome grains such as oats, quinoa, and basmati rice.

### *Detox Gently with Ghee*

A week of preparation is followed by three or four days of eating very simple: a mono diet of congee or Ayurvedic Tonic Kitchari (see page 238). In the morning, instead of breakfast, you drink an increasing amount of liquid ghee (starting with one tablespoon on day 1, increasing by one tablespoon each day until day 4), and then you do not eat anything until you are hungry. At bedtime on day 4, you take one to two tablespoons of castor oil in a little ginger tea, which will cleanse your bowels the next morning. That day, you rest, eat light, and slowly transition back into your regular diet, avoiding coffee, alcohol, sugar, and processed foods as long as you can.

## Resilience: Go Beyond Your Constitutional Stress Pattern in Three Easy Steps

The mind is a wonderful servant, but a terrible master.
—Proverb popularized by Robin Sharma in
*The Monk Who Sold His Ferrari*

Today, many of us find ourselves with never-ending to-do lists, rushing from one bullet point to the next, and often juggling many balls at once. "How are you?" has a unified answer: "Busy. Super busy." While being busy may no longer be as glorified as it was five or ten years ago, being stressed-out, frazzled, and short on time is still an accepted social norm. Fueled on sugar, adrenaline, and coffee, we rush through our daily lives only to collapse in the evening exhausted on the sofa, where we self-medicate with alcohol, chocolate, and binge-watching television or movies. The next morning we start all over again. Slowly but surely, we slouch toward depression and disease.

## Stress and Your Lymph

No matter what our stress pattern is, research shows clearly that if left unchecked, chronic stress can have a direct and devastating effect on our adrenals and other organ systems in our body, including the microbiome and cardiovascular and nervous systems.[4] Because both adrenaline and cortisol, and their metabolic waste products, free radicals, are extremely acidic in nature—and most of the body's immune and detox functions can only happen in an alkaline environment—it is our most important and primordial tissue, the lymphatic system, that is mostly affected by stress.

## We Are *Inflammageing*

As we discussed earlier, our lymphatic system (*rasa dhatu*) is the collective of our internal "waters" that provide juiciness, youth, and longevity when healthy, but promote disease, inflammation, and aging when congested, stagnant, and polluted. There is a term now that describes this pathological development: *inflammageing*.[5] Congested lymph (*rasa*) leads to a buildup of toxins (*ama*), accumulation of wastes, and disrupted metabolism of all the six bodily tissues (*dhatus*). The result: You start feeling subpar. You wake up tired and foggy, with stiff aching joints, dull skin or puffy eyes, and the need for caffeine and sugar to push through the day. Over time, your body's innate repair-and-rebound mechanisms break down, and belly fat, high cholesterol, and insulin resistance develop, leading to compromised immune function, autoimmune disease, depression, and cancer.

## Your Mind May Be the Most Critical Factor for Your Health

Throughout this book, we have seen that Ayurveda defines health not only as an absence of disease but as a positive state of vitality that encompasses all aspects of our being—body, mind, and soul. Those parts are not separate from each other but deeply interconnected. It is the mind—our thinking, sensing, and emotions—that forms the bridge between the physical and subtler aspects of our being. The mind and senses are our doorway to the world. How well we are connected to ourselves as well as the world at large depends on how skillfully we are using our mind. Do you remember the definition of health according to Ayurveda? One key aspect is *svastha*, or "being situated within yourself"—that is, knowing who you are. This applies to stress as well. Below we will look at how stress manifests differently in the various constitutional types. If you get to know your default pattern in stressful situations, you can take preventive action to buffer it when triggered.

### *Step 1. Know Your Evolutionary and Constitutional Stress Pattern*

In all living beings, stress triggers a sympathetic nervous system arousal that is referred to as our fight-flight-freeze response. Evolutionarily, when we were attacked by a tiger, we had the choice to fight back, run away, or pretend to be dead. These responses are wired into our DNA, but which of these three actions we (subconsciously) choose is not random. Ayurveda shows clearly that our stress reaction is largely dependent on our constitutional default pattern:

Movers run away (flight).
Transformers attack (fight).
Regenerators drop "dead" (freeze).

Knowing your evolutionary stress pattern is the first step toward breaking it.

**Movers: Anxious and Avoidant.** The light, airy, and sensitive nature of Movers tilts them under stress toward a flight response. Often provoked by overwork, multitasking, little sleep, and a diet high in raw, cold, or processed foods, the nervous system of Movers easily becomes ungrounded, frazzled, and overactive. This leads to mood swings, anxiety, worry, and scatteredness. Under stress, Movers start escaping responsibility, leaving tasks and projects unfinished, dropping difficult relationships, and avoiding clear communication and confrontation. Physically, insomnia, constipation, low appetite, and weight loss set in. If stress is prolonged for an extended period, Movers can spiral into adrenal depletion, burnout, and nervous breakdown.

**Transformers: Angry and Controlling.** Under stress, the hot and fiery nature of Transformers makes them prone to a fight response. Provoked by ambition, competition, perfectionism, and a diet high in inflammatory and acidic substances such as alcohol, meat, and coffee, the nervous system of Transformers easily tilts toward anger, irritability, short-temperedness, and impatience. Physically, typical Transformer stress signs are high blood pressure, headaches, acid reflux, ulcers, and skin disorders. Under prolonged stress, Transformers also become bossy, controlling, and aggressive toward others. Or they start self-judging and blaming when they fall short of their own self-imposed high standards. This can lead to self-loathing, depression, rage, self-harming, or addiction. If stress is prolonged for an extended period, Transformers are prone to developing autoimmune conditions or heart disease.

**Regenerators: Stuck and Lethargic.** While the heavy, dense, and slow nature of Regenerators makes them less prone to stress, once their nervous system is triggered, it usually responds with freezing. Fueled by a sedentary lifestyle, a lack of action, and a diet high in sugar, refined carbohydrates, and junk foods, the nervous system of Regenerators easily becomes stuck, lethargic, dull, and depressed. Procrastination and compensation through emotional eating or binge-watching TV series is common among Regenerators. Under pressure, they become paralyzed, stuck, and unable to act or move. If stress is prolonged for an extended period, Regenerators spiral into depression, obesity, diabetes, and thyroid disease.

### *Step 2. Learn to Buffer Your Constitutional Stress Pattern*

If you know your evolutionary stress pattern, you can more easily take measures to strengthen your nervous system and buffer your pattern of reactivity before you spiral down.

**Buffering the Flight Response in Movers.** Sensitive and high-strung Movers need to take special care to slow down, breathe, and protect their delicate nervous system from overstimulation and flight states. They benefit from warm and grounding foods, supportive friends, and calm environments, as well as regular mindfulness practices such as yoga, meditation, and breathing.

1. **Dial in routine.** Movers thrive on stability and routine. Creating a structured daily routine can provide you with a sense of grounding and stability and thus help to alleviate stress. Set yourself regular times for meals, sleep, exercise, and relaxation. Follow a consistent routine to help soothe your unpredictable moods and temperament and provide a sense of stability and control in times of stress.
2. **Slow down and take deep breaths.** Engaging in regular breathing practices can be highly beneficial for Movers. Such practices allow you to slow down, anchor your mind back to the present, reduce anxiety, and shift your nervous system into parasympathetic rest-and-relax mode. Alternate nostril breathing (*nadi shodhana*), humming bee breath (*brahmari*), or the Wim Hof breathing method are all fantastic ways of de-escalating a frantic Mover state. Make a point of starting your day with these practices to set the tone, especially when you know the rest of the day will be hectic and chaotic.
3. **Prioritize self-care.** Self-care is essential for maintaining balance during times of increased stress. Set aside time each day to engage in activities that nourish your body and mind. For Movers, gentle self-massage (*abhyanga*) with warm sesame oil is a must, as well as taking soothing baths or engaging in creative pursuits that bring joy and relaxation.
4. **Eat those fats.** The food that Movers consume plays a significant role in managing stress. Choose warm, grounding, and nourishing foods that counter your light and airy nature. Opt for cooked, warm meals with plenty of healthy fats (nuts and seeds, ghee, oily fish), whole grains, root vegetables, and mildly warming spices. Avoid excessive intake of caffeine, alcohol, raw foods, and cold drinks.
5. **Declutter and organize.** Movers are sensitive to their surroundings. Make sure to create a peaceful environment that supports your inner state of turmoil. Declutter and organize your workspace to promote a sense of order, clarity, and tranquility. It is also helpful to surround yourself with warm colors such as orange and

yellow, and soothing earthy or flowery aromatherapy scents such as lavender, patchouli, neroli, or jasmine.

**Buffering the Fight Response in Transformers.** The fiery Transformer types need to schedule regular breaks from pushing beyond limits and go-getter ambitions, and instead allow themselves to be playful and have a little fun. They benefit from alkaline and cooling foods and soothing activities in nature.

1. **Relax, play, and have fun.** Transformers tend to be driven and hyperfocused. This is why it is crucial for them to carve out dedicated time for play, relaxation, and fun. Engage in activities that help you unwind and release tension, such as yoga, dancing, or swimming. Turn up your playfulness through fun and shamelessly "unproductive" hobbies, such as playing music, singing, or doodling.
2. **Cool down that fire.** Transformers tend toward heat and intensity. To balance this, incorporate cooling practices into your daily routine. Opt for gentle, cooling exercises such as swimming or walking in nature. Drink plenty of room-temperature water infused with fresh mint and cucumbers throughout the day to stay hydrated. Apply cooling essential oils such as jasmine, sandalwood, or rose to your temples or wrists for a soothing and cooling effect.
3. **Favor greens.** Transformers benefit from an alkaline and cooling diet. Include a variety of fresh, seasonal, and predominantly plant-based foods. Favor sweet, bitter, and astringent tastes, such as leafy greens, sweet fruits, cucumbers, coconut water, and herbal teas. Minimize spicy, fried, and processed foods, as well as coffee and alcohol that can exacerbate heat, irritability, and inflammation.
4. **Loosen control and learn surrender.** Transformers can be passionate and fiery, which can sometimes lead to explosive emotional responses, especially if things do not turn out the way they want. Learn to cultivate surrender and a sense of nonattachment to outcomes. Remember that you cannot always be in the driver's

seat. Practice mindfulness and self-reflection to gain perspective and maintain calm and cool.

5. **Sweat it out.** Transformers benefit from regular physical activity to release excess heat, energy, stress, and tension. Ideally look for activities that are moderate to intense but noncompetitive, such as swimming, running, hiking, or yoga. Make sure to exercise in the early morning or late afternoon when the temperature is cooler. Balance intense workouts with calming practices such as restorative yoga or meditation.

**Buffering the Freeze Response in Regenerators.** Since their default pattern is stuckness and stagnation, Regenerators need activity and stimulation during stressful times. Daily physical exercise and vigorous breathing brings lightness and energy to mind, while avoiding overeating (especially breads and sweets) helps keep their body light and fluid.

1. **Break a sweat.** Regenerators benefit immensely from regular intense exercise to invigorate both body and mind, release stagnant energy, uplift mood, and reduce stress. Engage in activities that are energizing and stimulating, such as brisk walking, jogging, dancing, or more vigorous vinyasa or power yoga.
2. **Change it up.** Regenerators love routine and stability but introducing variety and stimulation can help combat freeze states and increase motivation. Change up your morning routine, explore new restaurants, meet different people, or travel to foreign places. Embrace change and try new experiences to invigorate your mind and prevent stagnation.
3. **Move that lymph.** Regenerators can benefit from morning routines (*dinacharya*) that increase energy, get rid of stagnation, and promote mental clarity, such as cold showers and dry-brushing. Incorporate breathing exercises that are invigorating and stimulating, such as skull-shining breath (*kapalabhati*) or bellows breath (*bhastrika*).
4. **Kick-start digestion and metabolism.** Regenerators tend toward sluggish digestion and metabolism, which can contribute

to feelings of heaviness and mental fog. Support your digestion by favoring warm, light, and easily digestible foods such as spicy soups, light broths, and steamed vegetables. Include spices such as ginger, chili, turmeric, and black pepper to enhance metabolism and kick-start agni. Avoid heavy, oily, or sugary foods that can exacerbate feelings of lethargy and stagnation.

5. **Uplift and stimulate.** Aromatherapy is a powerful tool that we can use to directly impact the mind and emotions. Choose essential oils with stimulating, uplifting, and invigorating scents, such as lemon, bergamot, peppermint, or eucalyptus. Diffuse these oils in your living or working spaces or dilute them in carrier oils for self-massage to promote alertness and clarity.

### *Step 3. Connect to the Brilliance of Your Constitutional Stress Pattern*

Our constitutional traits are always both a gift and challenge. Now that you have learned to navigate the challenges, you are ready to use your evolutionary stress pattern to your advantage by cultivating and harnessing its positive aspects.

**Movers Are Creative and Imaginative Problem-Solvers.** Movers can use some of their creative and adaptable personality traits to better deal with stressful situations. Your flight response can be positively channeled into

- Adaptability
- Instinctual sensitivity
- Creativity and imagination

**Adapt Quickly and Be Flexible.** Movers have a natural gift of speed, adaptability, and flexibility. This allows you to quickly adapt to new and changing conditions without taxing your nervous system. You do not resist that which you cannot change, which allows you to smoothly change direction or strategy.

**Tune In to Your Sensitivity.** Movers often have a heightened sensitivity to external stimuli. When confronted with stress, their nervous system is easily overwhelmed. Make this your advantage by listening to your inner sensor. Follow your instinctive desire to remove yourself when a situation becomes overwhelming. Seek a quiet and calm environment where you can recenter and calm down before you attempt a resolution. This way you avoid unnecessarily depleting your (already scarce) resources.

**Turn On Creativity and Imagination.** Movers possess a vibrant imagination and highly creative mind. In stressful situations, the flight response allows you to retreat and reevaluate. Often that helps you tap into your ability to think outside the box and find unconventional solutions. It also gives you the ability to visualize positive outcomes or even use artistic expression (writing, painting, music) as a form of therapy and stress release.

**Transformers Are Passionate and Assertive Problem-Solvers.** Transformers can use some of their type A personality traits to better deal with stressful situations. Their fight response can be positively channeled into

- Assertion and rising to the challenge
- Finding solutions
- Taking charge

**Be Assertive and Rise to the Challenge.** Transformers are known for their assertiveness and courage. You can easily turn on your power and shift your nervous system by perceiving stress as a challenge to be conquered. Rather than avoiding or giving up, your competitive spirit allows you to confront and tackle hurdles and conflict directly. Don't shy away from asserting yourself, set healthy boundaries, and do not give away your power and determination.

**Find Solutions.** Transformers possess superb analytical and problem-solving skills. Use your sharp intellect and strategic thinking to assess any stressful situation, identify potential solutions, and finally take logical and decisive action steps.

**Take Charge.** Transformers value control and autonomy. You know how to get a grip on a derailed situation rather than passively succumbing to chaos and catastrophe. Let your temperament allow you to take charge and lead. Thereby you actively influence the outcome and leverage your strong willpower to find (re)solutions.

**Regenerators Are Patient and Analytical Problem-Solvers.** Regenerators can use some of their stable and grounded personality traits to better deal with stressful situations. Their freeze response can be positively channeled into

- Buffering and resilience
- Reflective and aligned decision-making
- Thoughtful analysis and planning

**Buffering and Resilience.** Regenerators tend to have a stable personality and relaxed emotional state, which makes them less prone to being easily overwhelmed and frantic. Your calm and patient disposition prevents you from impulsive reactions that often exacerbate and escalate stressful situations. It also buys you time to process your emotions and respond in a more composed and appropriate manner. By pausing and gathering your energy, thus preserving your vital inner resources (*ojas*), you are less likely to deplete your adrenals.

**Reflective and Aligned Decision-Making.** The freeze response of Regenerators helps them tap into their intuitive nature. By stepping back and entering a state of stillness, you can not only assess the situation from a more detached perspective but also access your intuition and inner guidance. Pausing, observing, sensing, and reflecting helps you make more authentic, confident, and solid decisions.

**Thoughtful Analysis and Planning.** Regenerators usually excel at analysis and careful, strategic planning. The freeze response allows for thoughtful analysis, which solidifies your decisions. By taking your time and patiently waiting for the right moment to make your move, you are not wasting energy and resources and often score in the long run.

**Treating Stress and Mental Imbalance.** Health and healing in Ayurveda are always approached holistically, taking into account the physical, mental, emotional, and spiritual aspects of our being. The Western separation of mind and body does not exist in the East. Just like the heart-mind[6] is considered one organ, the body in Ayurveda is seen as nothing but a crystallization of the mind. That is why when we work with the mind, we always also work with the body; and when we work on the body, we always also address the mind. In this light, the first goal of an Ayurvedic approach to stress relief is always to first avoid subjecting the body to stressors and triggering a survival response through our food and lifestyle choices. If you have anxiety and trouble sleeping but are continuing to drink six cups of coffee a day, eating doughnuts for breakfast, and watching paranormal Netflix series at night, I can give you all the meditation practices and ashwagandha in the world and they will not be effective. If you have trouble with your mind, it is useful to first start with the *body basics* to plug you back into the infinite energy source of the universe.

In the previous section we explored some specific ways to work with our constitutional stress patterns. Here are some valuable general pointers for all constitutions:

### Top Five Anti-Stress Remedies for All Types

1. **Eat an anti-inflammatory diet.** Eat foods that are seasonal and suitable to your constitution or current state of imbalance. Base your diet largely on fresh fruits and vegetables, whole grains, legumes, and healthy fats. Avoid processed and fried foods, sugar, caffeine, and alcohol. Excellent brain and nervous system boosters are foods rich in omega-3 fatty acids, such as oily fish, nuts, seeds, and ghee from grass-fed cows. Seasonal eating gives the body an opportunity for rejuvenation, detoxification, and re-attunement.[7]
2. **Recalibrate your circadian and doshic rhythm.** Dinacharya, our morning and also daytime rituals that help dial us back into the flow of nature, are one of the best ways to de-stress the body and reestablish balance of the doshas and tissues. The closer you

orient your schedule to the natural flow already occurring in the environment, the better you prevent physiological stress, compromised metabolic activity, and inflammation. When it comes to supporting your brain and nervous system, there are two critical time periods. First, the Pitta or Transformer time between 10 p.m. and 2 a.m., when most of your body's metabolic cleansing, brain detox, and nervous system reboot is happening. So, getting to sleep before midnight and waking up around sunrise is crucial for (re)building physical and mental stress resilience. Another critical time for the nervous system is the Vata or Mover time between 2 p.m. and 6 p.m., when your body is demanding a significant amount of blood sugar to satisfy the higher energy needs of your mind. If you skipped lunch or ate just a salad or cold sandwich, you do not have enough energy to make it through the afternoon. The result? You feel tired and start craving that cookie, chocolate bar, or coffee, which in turn further destabilizes your blood sugar and stresses your body into acidity and your mind into overstimulation. A vicious cycle.

To avoid your midafternoon crash, eat a proper lunch with plenty of vegetables as well as healthy amounts of protein (beans, legumes, oily fish, meat) and fat (olive oil, ghee, nuts). This will sustain you through the afternoon and keep your blood sugar as well as your nervous system stable.

3. **Practice a self-care ritual.** Ayurveda emphasizes the importance of self-care routines for stress resilience. This can include morning rituals such as oil massage (*abhyanga*) for Movers, dry-brushing and a brisk morning walk for Regenerators, and breathing and spending time in nature for Transformers.
4. **Actively promote relaxation through sensory awareness.** Meditation is a powerful tool for reducing stress and promoting relaxation, and I highly recommend a daily sitting practice of at least fifteen to twenty minutes. However, I see in many of my clients that, especially during stressful times, this is the first practice that goes out the window. Many people find it immensely difficult to make time for a meditation practice when they are busy

or stressed, and they struggle to sit still and "shut off" their hyperstimulated minds.

If you find it difficult to implement a longer sitting meditation into your day, or if you do not have much experience with meditation and do not know where to start, I suggest starting with a practice called mindful sensory awareness, often also referred to as "orientation" because you orient yourself from the stories in your head back to the here and now. The method is deceivingly simple: You use your senses to bring you back to the present moment. Simply pause, take a deep breath, and choose one of your senses—sight, hearing, touch, taste, or smell. Intentionally focus on the sensations associated with the sense you have chosen. For example, if you pick sight, take a moment to observe your surroundings. Let your eyes wander around and notice the colors, shapes, and details around you. You can also let your eyes rest on anything you feel drawn to. If you pick hearing, listen to the quality, volume, and melody of different sounds in your environment and let your ears rest lightly and effortlessly on those sounds. It is important that you do this without getting caught up in thoughts, stories, labels, or judgments. This practice takes no more than one to two minutes but immediately plugs you back into the here and now.

5. **Use adaptogenic herbs.** Ayurveda has powerful adaptogenic herbs such as ashwagandha, tulsi, and licorice to support the body and mind at times of increased physical or mental stress. In this chapter, we will see exactly how these rejuvenating herbs work.

## Long Before Biohacking: Rasayana— Ayurveda's Time-Tested Longevity and Antiaging Secrets

If aging means loss of juice—think leaves drying up, twigs becoming brittle, or our skin wrinkling and sagging—then its antidote is *rasayana.* Often translated as "rejuvenation," literally *rasayana* means "the path of juice" (*rasa*, "juice, essence"; *ayana*, "path, journey"). Rasayana foods, herbs, and therapies help guide the body away from disease, weakness, and premature aging toward a path of health, juiciness, vitality, and longevity.

### *The Ancient Elixirs of Immortality: Soma and Amrit*

The concept of immortality has been a topic of fascination for humans throughout history and has been explored in various myths, legends, and religious texts. In Hindu mythology, *amrit* (*a*, "not"; *mriyut*, "death") is a divine nectar and the elixir of immortality. Amrit is said to have been produced during one of the epic battles of the *Mahabharata*, the churning of the ocean of milk.[8] The ancient precursor to the Hindu amrit may be the *soma* juice of Vedic mythology. The *Rigveda*, one of the oldest sacred texts in the world, contains many hymns dedicated to soma and its powerful effects. Presently we do not know how the Vedic people extracted this soma juice, but there are some indications that soma was actually an intoxicating and hallucinogenic plant (similar to ayahuasca) used in the rituals by the Vedic priests to enter into a state of revery and communicate with gods and ancestors.

### *Ayurveda Invented the Concept of Antiaging*

While the global antiaging industry is a multi-billion-dollar business and one of the fastest growing markets, the concept behind antiaging—rejuvenation and longevity therapies—has been an established branch of Ayurvedic medicine for thousands of years. Treatments aimed at strengthening the body as well as restoring and preserving health, juice, and youthfulness using herbs and minerals were considered so vital that it evolved into its own branch as part of the eight branches of Ayurveda (Ashtanga Ayurveda). One of the reasons being probably that originally Ayurveda was the medicine for royals; to ensure long life of the king and secure healthy offspring, rasayana therapies were crucial.

### *Rejuvenation Is More Than Popping Pills*

Today, the market of superfoods, adaptogenic herbs, and medicinal mushrooms is booming. Stressed out, overworked, sleep-deprived, and exhausted, many of us feel in need of "juice." While it may be tempting to add energy-boosters such as ashwagandha, cordyceps, or ginseng to your routine, traditional systems of medicine, such as Chinese medicine or Ayurveda, hold that rejuvenation and tonification are more than just popping a few pills. It is a systematic process of cleansing, recalibrating, and rebuilding.

### *First Detox, Then Rejuvenate*

According to the classical texts, before beginning any rejuvenation therapies, the body must be cleansed. Just as you cannot dye a stained cloth (the color will not take hold), so you cannot rejuvenate and rebuild a body full of ama (toxins). We could say that the purpose of panchakarma, the famous Ayurvedic series of cleansing procedures, is mainly to prepare the body for rasayana, or rejuvenation. After the cleansing, you can start a period of rejuvenation, often removed from daily life and stressors, where you are guided to avoid intoxicants such as tobacco and alcohol; retreat to a quiet, calm, nurturing space; consume simple foods predominantly in the sweet taste (the most nourishing of the six tastes), including ghee, milk, and honey; and use appropriate rasayana herbs and supplements. For those not able to undergo a full panchakarma and retreat to the mountains or countryside for extended periods, a shorter fast or cleanse as outlined earlier is a perfect priming and preparation before starting rejuvenating herbs and supplements.

### *The Long Track Record of Rasayana Herbs*

Without classifying them as adaptogens per se, Chinese medicine and Ayurveda have been using tonic herbs for thousands of years to support overall strength and well-being, tone particular organ (systems), and heal a wide variety of ailments. The term *adaptogen* was initiated much later, in the mid-twentieth century, by the Russian scientists Nikolai Lazarov and Israel Breckman. They started exploring chemical compounds that could help promote health by increasing the state of what they referred to as "nonspecific resistance to stress." The definition they came up with was that to be considered an adaptogen, an herb or plant substance must

- Be nontoxic at normal doses
- Support the body's ability to cope with stress, no matter whether physical, environmental, or mental-emotional
- Help the body return to a state of stability by normalizing bodily function on a wide range of organs and tissues

### *The Market for Adaptogens Is Booming*

Ever since then, much research has been conducted on various adaptogens and their health benefits. Today, adaptogens are considered a class of very intelligent herbs that can modulate our body's reaction to stress and help us better adapt to stressors. Supporting many essential processes in the body, adaptogens excel at improving mood, balancing hormones, fighting fatigue, and boosting the immune system. Traditionally they were cooked into teas, milk, or medicinal broths, but today they are also found in capsules or powders that people add to smoothies and shakes.

## My Top Three Ayurvedic Rasayanas or Adaptogens

1. **Ashwagandha:** a supremely nourishing root that excels at building muscle strength and stamina, and alleviates anxiety and depression
2. **Tulsi:** a sacred type of basil found around many temples in India that boosts immunity and lung function, alleviates stress, and decreases anxiety
3. **Shilajit:** a black mineral pitch that oozes out of rocks in the Himalayas and modulates inflammation, aging, and cognitive decline

### *Ashwagandha (Withania somnifera)*

Ashwagandha is one of the most important and versatile Ayurvedic herbs. It is a tonic but not as sweet, cooling, and heavy as most rejuvenating herbs. Being lighter and warmer, it is also useful for Regenerator types. While ashwagandha is mainly known as a male rejuvenating tonic (it literally means "smelling like a horse"), it can be used for both sexes as a supreme strength-building herb. Ashwagandha is superb in all conditions of weakness, depletion, and stress since it promotes anabolic growth, helping to build both muscle and strength.[9] Taken in the morning, it will energize and sustain; taken at night before bed, it will help promote deep and rejuvenating sleep. Recent additional research shows its benefit in cancer treatment through immune-modulating and cytotoxic activity.[10]

**How to Use.** As a tonic, ashwagandha is traditionally cooked into milk with a pinch of ginger or cinnamon to support assimilation. However, you can also cook it into a plant-based milk, such as hemp or almond milk, or use it with plain hot water. Use a half teaspoon once or twice a day.

### *Tulsi (Ocimum sanctum)*

Tulsi, or holy basil, is one of the most revered sacred plants in India and is frequently used in various Hindu rituals and ceremonies. Nearly every Indian home has a tulsi plant at the entrance or in the courtyard to purify, protect, and uplift the environment. In Hindu mythology, Tulsi is a goddess and worshipped as a symbol of purity, devotion, and protection. Taken internally, tulsi helps cope with stress, promotes mental clarity, uplifts mood, and supports rejuvenation.[11] Because tulsi is pungent and warming, it is a wonderful tea for fall and winter, as well as for flu season. It warms the body, increases circulation, boosts and cleanses lymph (*rasa*), removes excess congestion and mucous from the lungs, and boosts prana or qi (vital life force) levels.

**How to Use.** You can buy tulsi as dried leaves or powder and brew it as a delicious tea, steeping one teaspoon of leaves in one cup of boiling water for eight to ten minutes. In fall and winter, I like to combine tulsi with ginger; in spring, for extra liver support, with nettle and mint; and in summer or during times of mental-emotional stress, I add rose.

### *Shilajit (Asphaltum punjabianum)*

Shilajit is a highly sought-after dark mineral substance that oozes out of rocks in the high mountain range of the Himalayas. Not a plant per se but rather an amalgamate, it is created when plants slowly decompose over centuries into the rocks, merging with the rock minerals to form a sticky, tar-like substance. Eventually, stimulated by the pressure of summer heat, shilajit is squeezed out of the rocks and ready to be harvested. While the Sanskrit word *shilajit* literally means "destroyer of weakness," the substance is often also called "blood of the mountains," directly referring to this unusual formation.

**Uniquely Detoxifying and Rejuvenating.** Highly esteemed and traditionally used in Ayurveda and Tibetan medicine for thousands of years as a supreme antiaging substance, shilajit has several exceptional features. First, it is rich in many trace minerals such as silica and iron, and it contains fulvic and humic acid. These antioxidant and anti-inflammatory compounds are formed when plant material breaks down over long periods of time. Second, shilajit is both an effective detoxifier—it purifies blood, and removes Kapha, fat, and accumulations from the body—and a supreme rejuvenator. It strengthens the natural function of the immune system, supports the kidneys, and fortifies bones.[12]

**Shilajit Protects Against Neurodegeneration.** As a rejuvenating and antiaging substance, shilajit also tones the reproductive organs, boosts testosterone levels, and revitalizes libido, all while promoting longevity and a youthful glow. Considering its high mineral content and ability to support many tissues, it is no surprise that shilajit is considered an adaptogen that helps the body cope with stress by supporting adrenals and thyroid, boosting mitochondrial function, and stabilizing the nervous system. Recent research also examines the use of shilajit for cognitive and neurodegenerative disorders associated with aging, such as Alzheimer's and dementia.[13] Last but not least, shilajit is also known as a *yogavahi*, or "catalyst" (*yoga*, "uniting, joining"; *vahi*, "vehicle, carrier"), because of its ability to carry and drive nutrients deep into the body so they can work most effectively. As such, it is often used as a catalyst in formulations with other herbs to enhance their effectiveness.

**How to Use.** Because it is a dense and sticky substance, shilajit is often available in capsules and tablets rather than powder form. The regular dose is one to two tablets once or twice daily with warm water.

# Part Three

## Living Ayurveda 2.0: Your Journey

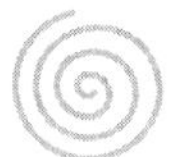  

# 7

## Baseline: Let's Take Inventory

Far from being just another diet or weight loss program, the journey you are about to take is just the beginning of your life with Ayurveda. Over the course of several weeks, I will guide you step by step to walk your way (back) to health, vitality, and wellness. As I promised at the beginning of this book, this is not about deprivation or adding more bullet points to your life that is already stressful and overwhelming. Rather, it is a coming home to the innate wisdom and resources you already have within yourself—an intuitive and immensely rewarding stroll through the beautiful and rich landscape of an Ayurvedic way of living. We do this by activating the three most crucial factors for health and longevity: circadian returning, metabolic optimization, and lymphatic cleansing.

### How Far Are You from Your Full Potential?

We have previously seen that while our constitution (*prakriti*) never changes, the doshas are constantly subject to change. Time of day, season, lifestyle, food, and emotions can all influence and cause the doshic balance to change. Emotional and physical health in Ayurveda is never an absolute state but a constant dance to readjust to be as close to your original genetic blueprint as possible. It is about realigning yourself with your innate nature. Over time you learn to read the clues to your imbalances and can take necessary measures to restore harmony. For example, when I find myself ungrounded, anxious, and with dry skin, maybe even slightly constipated, I know that my Vata dosha is out of balance and that I may need to focus on warm, cooked foods, a regular routine, and rest to regain balance.

One of the strongest assets of Ayurveda is its concept of radical bio-individuality. Rather than addressing symptoms and treating them with a one-size-fits-all approach, Ayurveda focuses on the individual with their unique metabolic needs, digestive strength, level of toxicity, and mental-emotional state. While this is a no-brainer and easily achieved in my practice, where I work with clients individually, to do this in a book read by thousands of (metabolically) unique individuals is a different ball game. This is why, before you start your Ayurveda 2.0 journey of exploration and recalibration, I invite you to first take inventory of your current state of metabolic strength versus imbalance. We will do this by assessing the three most important factors in disease formation, according to Ayurveda:

1. Your doshic imbalance (*vikriti*)
2. Your gut health (*agni*)
3. Your level of endotoxicity (*ama*)

Based on your imbalance, the strength of your gut, and the level of ama in your body, you determine which track of this journey is more suitable to your needs and which doshic imbalance you will mainly work on during your journey toward health.

---

## Assess Your Imbalances (*Vikriti*)

Which one of the following symptoms have you been experiencing recently? Please check all the boxes that apply:

Vata

- ☐ My mind is jumpy and scattered. I have difficulty concentrating and completing tasks.
- ☐ I feel anxious, stressed, and overwhelmed. I am "tired but wired."
- ☐ I have trouble switching my mind off at night. It is difficult for me to fall and/or stay asleep.
- ☐ My daily routine (exercise, mealtimes, self-care) has been erratic.

- ☐ My appetite and digestion have been variable, with gas, bloating, and irregular bowel movements.
- ☐ My weight fluctuates. I can easily lose my appetite when I am stressed and anxious.
- ☐ My skin is always dry, no matter how much I moisturize.
- ☐ My nails and hair are brittle; my joints are popping and cracking.

Total: ______________

Pitta

- ☐ I can be easily irritated, impatient, critical, and judgmental of others.
- ☐ In my work, I push myself (and others) hard to achieve perfection.
- ☐ I am (in)tense and competitive. I have a difficult time relaxing and easing off.
- ☐ I feel warm and I sweat easily, even when others around me feel comfortable.
- ☐ My skin is reddish, sensitive, and easily irritated and inflamed.
- ☐ My appetite is high, and I am thirsty all the time.
- ☐ After spicy or fried foods, I can get a burning sensation or acidity in my stomach.
- ☐ My bowel movements are on the loose side, even diarrhea sometimes.

Total: ______________

Kapha

- ☐ I am overweight and have a sluggish metabolism.
- ☐ I feel puffy and swollen, especially in my face, fingers, and ankles.
- ☐ In the morning, my tongue is puffy, with a thick white coating.
- ☐ When I am stressed or emotionally upset, I tend to crave and overeat sweets and refined carbohydrates such as bread and pasta.

- ☐ I have a hard time getting out of bed in the morning and need a nap after lunch.
- ☐ I need coffee to feel awake and clear my brain fog.
- ☐ I feel congested, and when sick, I can easily develop mucous in my body and lungs.
- ☐ I feel lethargic and too lazy to move, exercise, or do anything.

Total: ____________

Results

If you checked any boxes under each of the three doshas listed, you have an imbalance in that particular dosha. For most of us, there is one dosha that is significantly more imbalanced than the others, but it is also possible that you may show imbalances in two or even all of the doshas.

< 2 Mild Imbalance

2–4 Moderate Imbalance

> 4 Strong Imbalance

## Assess Your Gut Function (*Agni*)

Here is a quick assessment tool for checking your current digestive health (*agni*). On the first round, in chapter 5, you answered according to your general digestive tendencies to determine your overall digestive and metabolic strength (*agni dosha*). Now, on the second round, please answer strictly according to your *current* or relatively *recent* digestive symptoms.

1. How do you feel after eating a meal these days?
   a. I feel satiated and full of energy.
   b. I feel bloated or gassy.
   c. Usually good, but if the food is too spicy or oily, I can get heartburn, acidity, or reflux.

d. I feel heavy, stuffed, and sleepy after meals. My energy goes down.

2. How is your current appetite and hunger level?
   a. It is pretty regular.
   b. My appetite varies every day. If I am busy, I forget to eat. Often my eyes are bigger than my stomach.
   c. My appetite is strong. I am almost always hungry and can eat big portions.
   d. My appetite is low. I can feel full for a long time after eating. I eat more for pleasure and comfort than actual hunger.

3. What happens if you skip a meal?
   a. I can easily skip a meal and feel totally fine.
   b. I need to eat more frequently. If I forget to eat, I can easily get lightheaded and hypoglycemic.
   c. I hate skipping meals. I get cranky, irritable, and (h)angry.
   d. I can easily skip meals and feel much better if I eat less.

4. Which foods tend to bother you the most these days?
   a. I can eat everything and digest it well.
   b. I get gassy and bloated with raw salads; beans and lentils; and cruciferous vegetables such as broccoli, cabbage, and cauliflower.
   c. If I eat fried, oily, or spicy foods, I get heartburn and acid reflux.
   d. I get sleepy and/or congested after eating sweets, refined carbs, and dairy products such as cheese, yogurt, or ice cream.

5. How is your elimination?
   a. Normal. I have a well-formed bowel movement every morning.
   b. Irregular. I have constipation with dry and small pellet stools.
   c. Frequent. I have two to three bowel movements per day, on the soft or liquid side.
   d. Regular. My stools are heavy and bulky. Rarely, there also can be mucous in the stool.

Now count how many a, b, c, and d answers you got.

a = ________

b = ________

c = ________

d = ________

Remember that agni has four clinical states. It can be perfectly balanced (*sama*); erratic and irregular (*vishama*); burning intensely and sharp (*tikshna*); or low, dull, and sluggish (*manda*).

a. Sama agni: If you scored mostly **a** answers, congratulations. You have perfect digestion, or sama agni. Currently your digestion, absorption, and elimination are all normal, and you can digest any type of food in any season without adverse signs and symptoms.
b. Vishama agni: If you scored mostly **b** answers, you currently have an erratic and irregular digestive fire, or vishama agni. Often due to the cold and mobile qualities of Vata, agni can fluctuate and become erratic, producing irregular appetite, variable digestion, bloating, gas, constipation, and colicky pain.
c. Tikshna agni: If you scored mostly **c** answers, you have a hot, sharp, and acidic digestive system, or tikshna agni. Through the hot and sharp quality of Pitta dosha, agni can become intense and cause intense hunger and thirst, a need for large quantities of food, heartburn and acid reflux, or diarrhea.
d. Manda agni: If you scored mostly **d** answers, you have dull, slow, and sluggish digestion and metabolism, or manda agni. The heavy, slow, and dull quality of Kapha dosha can extinguish agni and make it work subpar. Even when fasting or eating very little, because of manda agni, you can put on weight. There is heaviness in the stomach, loss of appetite, fullness, and sleepiness after meals.

## Assess Your Level of Endotoxicity (*Ama*)

In order to assess if you have toxins as a result of improper digestion, please review the list below and checkmark each symptom that applies to you currently.

- ☐ Lack of appetite
- ☐ Lack of taste
- ☐ Bad breath
- ☐ Thick white or yellow coating on the tongue in the morning
- ☐ Smelly gas and stools
- ☐ Sticky stools that stain the toilet
- ☐ Indigestion
- ☐ Chronic mucous or congestion (sinuses/lungs)
- ☐ Feeling of heaviness and lethargy
- ☐ Brain fog
- ☐ Smelly sweat and/or urine
- ☐ Joint inflammation and pain
- ☐ Dull aches and pains (especially whole body and roots of hair)
- ☐ Skin issues such as acne, pimples, rashes

Total:

0–1 Bravo. Your level of toxicity is zero or very low and mostly limited to your digestive system.

2–3 There is some level of ama in your digestive system and possibly also in your systemic circulation.

> 3 You have ama in your digestive system, systemic circulation, and possibly even lodged in your deeper tissues.

If you have marked more than one symptom on the list above, it is likely that you have some ama in your system. More than three checkmarks means your body is in need of some deeper cleansing and a digestive reboot. Please don't worry; this is just your starting point. The deeper cleansing and rebooting will happen naturally as you progress through the different stages.

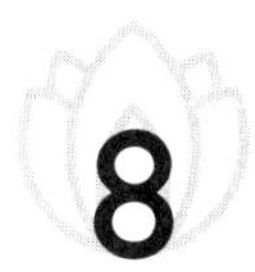

# 8

# The Ayurveda 2.0 Journey

## Your Healing Journey

Now that you are ready to set out on your healing journey, there are essentially two tracks you can take:

1. Slow Mojo (Beginner): eighteen weeks
2. Turbo Track (Advanced): nine weeks

To assess your complete health status, please check the following table:

| **Assessment Results** | | |
|---|---|---|
| Vikriti Test | > 2 in one, two, or three doshas | 1–2 in one or two doshas only |
| Gut Health | vishama, manda, or tikshna agni | sama, vishama, tikshna, or manda agni |
| Ama Test | > 3<br>Ama is lodged in the digestive system, systemic circulation, and deeper tissues. | 0–1<br>Your level of toxicity is zero or very low and mostly limited to your digestive system. |
| **TRACK** | **SLOW MOJO** | **TURBO TRACK** |

**Slow Mojo (Beginner):** If you are new to Ayurveda and/or have scored higher in terms of imbalance, gut function, and ama, then I highly recommend you take it slow and enjoy the ride. Remember, fast is not necessarily better. I propose you take at least two to three weeks for each step of the program and about six to nine weeks for each stage.

This ensures that the changes you implement will stick and become as automatic and easy as brushing your teeth. For the changes to do their magic and alter your physiology, they need time. Remember, each stage builds on top of the next. If you aren't plugged back into the matrix of circadian wiring (stage 1, Flow), your digestion, metabolic activity, and hormones will be difficult to balance (stage 2, Transform). Similarly, if your diet is off and you are not assimilating nutrients properly, we cannot work on lymphatic cleansing and a nervous system reboot (stage 3, Regenerate). Each stage lays the foundation for the next so we can activate your body's innate healing power.

**Turbo Track (Advanced):** You are ready for this track if you are already familiar with Ayurveda and have been practicing some of the daily routines, such as tongue scraping or oil pulling, for at least six months; and/or if your imbalances and ama levels are all in the lower range. Building on the foundation of habits and health you already have, you will be able to move through the program quickly, taking only one week for each step, or three weeks for each of the three stages—nine weeks in total. Since you are probably already fairly healthy and paying attention to your diet, exercise, and anti-stress routines, your goal will be to go one step further. You will refine your vitality and resilience and fortify your body's inbuilt longevity switch.

Are you ready?

## Hack 1: Flow—Sync with Nature Through Circadian Retuning

In this first step of our journey, you plug back into the matrix by resetting your circadian rhythm and attuning to the doshic waves throughout day and night. This starts optimizing the way you Flow.

### *Week 1: Scrape, Hydrate, Swap, Digital Detox, Perfect Poop*

During your first week, you start to support your body's inherent circadian rhythm by implementing a few powerful Ayurvedic morning (*dinacharya*) and evening (*ratricharya*) routines.

#### Morning Routine

- **Scrape:** Add tongue scraping to your morning practice, right before or after brushing your teeth. This will not only eliminate excess toxin (*ama*) buildup after detoxification at night but also stimulate a set of acupressure points on your tongue connected to your vital organs.
- **Hydrate:** Instead of coffee or tea, start your day with Morning Lemon-Honey Water (see page 231). The lemon cleanses the liver, stimulates the intestines, and helps alkalinize the body. Honey scrapes excess Kapha, mucous, and fat from the body but can be omitted if you are (intermittent) fasting or have a lot of dryness in your body.

  *Note:* According to Ayurveda, honey turns toxic when heated above 40°C. So make sure your water is warm and not hot before you add the honey.
- **Swap:** If you are used to starting your day with coffee, switch to enjoying your cup after breakfast, or at least an hour and a half to two hours after waking, to let the body's inbuilt wake-up mechanism run its course before you interfere.[1] Also, do not drink caffeinated beverages (coffee, tea, cacao) after 2 p.m. Since the half-life of caffeine—the amount of time it takes for the body to process just half—is usually five hours, but can also take up to nine hours, an afternoon latte or post-dinner espresso can deeply interfere with your deep-sleep cycle and interrupt your circadian rhythm. The ideal time to consume your coffee is in between breakfast and lunch, ideally before noon.

#### Evening Ritual

We discussed in the first part of the book that your evening greatly determines how easily you get out of bed in the morning and how smooth your day flows. Heavy or late-night dinners, excessive alcohol, or staying up past midnight are all habits that can compromise your body's ability to detoxify and regenerate overnight. So, this week, please implement the following:

- **Digital detox:** Switch off electronics (TV, phone, computer) by 9 p.m. at the latest. Electronics such as smartphones, tablets, and computer screens emit blue light, which can suppress the production of melatonin, a hormone that regulates sleep. Blue-light exposure in the evening can trick your brain into thinking it is still daytime, making it harder to fall asleep and disrupting your circadian rhythm. Engaging with electronic devices at night also overstimulates your mind before bed rather than priming it for winding down and deep rest.
- **Perfect poop:** It is vital to have a regular elimination in the morning. To start regulating your bowels and help detoxify the gut, please start taking the supreme Ayurvedic bowel cleanser and rejuvenating formula Triphala at a dose of a half teaspoon of powder or two capsules at bedtime with hot water. If you cannot find Triphala, you can use psyllium husks—a plant fiber—at the dose of one teaspoon in a big glass of water at bedtime.

### *Week 2: Early Rise, Swish, Swap, "Adieu, Night Owls"*

After the circadian switch last week, this week is all about aligning your internal fire (*agni*) with the natural cycle of the sun, the external fire.

#### Morning Routine

- **Early rise:** We are diurnal beings, so getting up before or around sunrise is vital for circadian fine-tuning. If right now you are waking up at 8 a.m. or 9 a.m., start adjusting your wake-up time gradually to move closer to between 6 a.m. and 7 a.m. Not only will this give you more time in the morning for your cleansing and centering routines, but it also helps readjust your circadian rhythm and support your sleep at night more effectively.
- **Swish:** After tongue scraping, add five minutes of oil pulling with plain coconut oil or a special medicated oil pulling oil. Slowly increase day by day up to fifteen minutes.

### Midday

- **Swap:** Make brunch or lunch (between 11 a.m. and 1 p.m.) your biggest meal and dinner lighter. Your digestive and metabolic capacity (*agni*) is stronger during the day than in the evening, so eating a good lunch and a smaller dinner is much more supportive for digestion, weight, and more restful sleep. You will notice that it is much easier to get out of bed if you eat a smaller and earlier dinner.

This week, try at least two of the following recipes from the recipe section:

- Lunch: Freestyle Lunch Bowl (according to your imbalance, or *vikriti*)
- Dinner: Sup(p)er Soups

### Evening Ritual

- **"Adieu, Night Owls":** Adjust your bedtime in increments of fifteen minutes each day until you arrive at 10 p.m. (if right now you go to bed way past midnight, then aim at least for 11 p.m.). If you have trouble sleeping, please experiment with some of the sleep hacks in the nighttime ritual (*ratricharya*) section, such as
  - Warm oil massage for the feet (*padabhyanga*)
  - Relaxing bedtime breathwork, such as nadi shodhana
  - A guided evening meditation, such as yoga nidra
  - A cup of Deep-Sleep Tonic (see page 231)

## *Week 3: Move, Unwind, Close the Kitchen*

This week, we are going one step further by not only attuning to the circadian waning of day and night but also connecting to the larger seasonal cycles that happen as the sun moves around the earth.

### Morning Routine

- **Move:** Add ten minutes of morning movement and stretching. If you can do it outside, even better, since sunlight or daylight right after getting up primes your sleep hormones at night.

**General.** Attune to the season you are currently in. Each season brings with it its own unique energy and character. The better we align ourselves with the rhythm and qualities of each season, the less likely we are to become imbalanced. You may already be doing some of this intuitively. If not, you can remind yourself of the energetic pattern and theme of each season by referring to the section on seasonal routines (*ritucharya*).

**Spring:** As the sun returns after the long, dark winter months, we tune in to the energy of *new beginnings* and growth.
**Summer:** We naturally tap into the energy of abundance, *passion*, and joy.
**Fall:** We embrace the energy of change, *letting go*, and transformation.
**Winter:** We tune in to the energy of *rest* and introspection.

### Evening Ritual

- **Unwind:** After work, take ten minutes to stretch and breathe. This will help you unwind and transition from "work" mode to fully arriving at home. I often put on a favorite song and dance or shake to let go of the accumulated stressors of the day that are often lodged in our muscles and tissues.
- **Close the Kitchen:** Close the kitchen by 7 p.m. at the latest. Don't eat anything afterward, until breakfast the next morning. This starts a gentle Ayurvedic version of what is commonly referred to as intermittent fasting (IF).

  Breakfast is ideally around:
  - 8 a.m.–9 a.m. for Movers, which means you are fasting for thirteen to fourteen hours.
  - 9 a.m.–10 a.m. for Transformers, which means you are fasting for fourteen to fifteen hours.
  - 11 a.m.–1 p.m. for Regenerators, which means you are fasting for sixteen to eighteen hours.

## Hack 2: Transform—Undiet by Optimizing Digestion and Metabolism

### *Week 1: Smart Eating, Cut Cold, Agni Boost*

According to Ayurveda, your digestive and metabolic power (*agni*) is one of the most important factors for health and longevity. During the next few weeks, you will focus on reigniting your agni through a few simple yet highly effective and practical hacks that you can easily apply in your daily life. In the first week, your focus is on eliminating all the things that slow down your digestive power, especially cold foods and drinks, as well as incompatible food combinations.

- **Smart eating:** Start following the two most important Ayurvedic food combining rules. First, fresh fruit should not be mixed with any other foods, especially dairy products. Fruit digests very fast and thus should always be eaten alone. Let go of fruit-based smoothies or yogurt with fresh fruit. Second, two different animal products at one meal are very difficult to digest, so avoid drinking a latte with your omelet or eating fish or meat cooked in a cream sauce.

  Don't eat:
  - Fruit + anything
  - Dairy (milk, cheese, yogurt, cream, kefir) + eggs, meat, fish
- **Cut cold:** Avoid cold foods and iced drinks, especially with meals. This means food straight from the refrigerator as well as ice cream or iced drinks such as cold kombucha, iced lattes, or iced tea. Cold foods and drinks greatly weaken digestion. Just think about adding ice cubes to a pot of rice that is cooking. What would happen? The cooking process would be halted and a significant amount of energy would be needed to heat the water back to boiling.

  Instead, I encourage you to try *garam pani*, the Ayurvedic hot water cure, which is a fantastic way to cleanse and hydrate the digestive tract, stimulate the lymphatic system, and strengthen agni. Traditionally you would boil water in a glass or stainless-steel pot for at least ten minutes, which changes the subtle properties of the water and makes it easier to assimilate. If this is not possible or practical, you can use regular boiled water and sip on it every twenty to thirty minutes, with or in between meals.

- **Agni boost:** For a deeper digestive reboot and to start eliminating toxins (*ama*), start sipping on a cup of Tame the Flame Tea (see page 226) daily after or in between meals. Also start adding spices according to the result of your agni test.
    - **Vishama agni:** Add a quarter teaspoon of Tame the Flame Spice (Hingvasthak Churna) (see page 227) under your tongue after your main meal of the day.
    - **Tikshna agni:** Chew a half teaspoon of Happy Belly Spice (see page 228) after your main meal of the day.
    - **Manda agni:** Eat a slice of Ayurvedic Ginger Pickle (see page 226) ten minutes before your main meal of the day.

### *Week 2: Balance, Nourish, Raw Swap, Simplify*

This week we go one step further to personalize your diet according to your individual doshic imbalance (*vikriti*). And we start to incorporate some gut-healing recipes to rebuild the lining of your digestive tract.

- **Balance:** Adjust your diet according to the results of your vikriti (imbalance) quiz. If your Pitta is elevated, you will follow a Pitta-balancing foods list; if Vata is high, you will follow a Vata-balancing list. If you are perfectly balanced, then adjust your diet according to the season. Please refer to the seasonal or doshic food lists in part two or start shopping at a local farmers market, where you find produce that is in season.
- **Nourish:** To start rebuilding your gut, make sure that this week you add one cup of Gut-Healing Marrow Bone (or Chicken) Broth or Gut-Healing Vegan Miso Broth (see recipes section) daily. You can drink these by themselves or use them as a base for soups.
- **Raw swap:** Stop eating raw foods (salads or raw fruits) in the evening after sunset, when your digestion is weaker. Lunchtime or early-dinner salads are fine in spring and summer, when the weather is warmer.
- **Simplify:** Stick to two or three meals per day. Avoid snacking in

between meals. This makes sure that the previous meal is fully digested before new food enters the stomach. Generally, Movers do better with three meals per day, while Transformers and Regenerators do great with only two meals per day.

### *Week 3: Prana Boost, Savor, Good Bugs*

Now we are ready to move even one step further. Avoiding leftovers, make sure that your food brims with life energy. As you start to repopulate your gut with beneficial bacteria, you make your agni more resilient in the long run.

- **Prana boost:** Prepare your meals fresh as much as possible, avoiding leftovers. Fresh foods are rich in prana, the vital life force or energy present in living things. As time passes, the prana in food diminishes and the energetic qualities of the food change. Bacteria and other microorganisms can multiply in leftover food, leading to the accumulation of toxins, or ama.
- **Enjoy:** Take time and pleasure to eat and chew your food well. When you eat, don't do anything else, such as checking your phone, working, walking, or driving.
- **Good bugs:** Make or buy Probiotic Beet Kvass (see page 233) or any lacto-fermented vegetable you enjoy (such as kimchi or sauerkraut). Take one glass of kvass or one or two tablespoons of fermented veggies with lunch or dinner for superb probiotic support. Alternatively, one capsule of a wide-spectrum probiotic in the morning on an empty stomach is also effective at boosting beneficial gut bacteria. After you have finished the complete nine- or eighteen-week journey, you can also use homemade kefir or yogurt for probiotic support now that you can digest dairy well.

## Hack 3: Regenerate: Dial Into Longevity by Developing Physical and Mental Resilience

Now that you are attuned to the daily and seasonal cycles as well as supported by a steady-burning internal fire (digestion and metabolism), you are ready to enter the last phase of our program: rebuilding and regeneration.

### *Week 1: Lymph Boost, Eliminate, Adrenal Prime*

This week is all about decongesting your lymphatic system. Remember, the healthier your lymph, your waste-removal system, the more resilient your body and the calmer your mind.

#### Morning Routine

- **Lymph boost:** To start supporting the lymphatic tissue (*rasa*), implement a hot-cold shower therapy. For the details regarding contrast shower or hydrotherapy, please refer to the section on morning routines (*dinacharya*). In general, I recommend doing a contrast shower in fall and winter and a cold shower only in summer or if you are a Transformer type with abundant internal heat and fire.

  Step 1: You can still take a warm or hot shower, but just make sure to finish your shower cold for thirty seconds or up to one minute.

  Step 2: For deeper benefits, start alternating hot and cold water for three rounds in total. One round is one-minute hot water, followed by thirty seconds or one minute cold water.

  *Tip:* If this is still very difficult for you, you can at least use cold water to finish off on your arms and legs (working your way from your extremities to your core).

  *Caution:* Please skip cold water if you are sick, have indigestion, or are menstruating.
- **Breathe:** Before or after your contrast shower, practice ten minutes of Wim Hoff breathing to energize your body and strengthen your nervous system. If you are pressed for time in the morning, you can also practice alternate nostril breathing (*nadi shodhana*) in the evening before bed. This harmonizes the left and right side of your brain and balances sympathetic and parasympathetic nervous function.

### General

- **Eliminate:** Cut out refined sugar, artificial sweeteners, dairy, and gluten for at least three weeks, starting this week. This will help lower inflammation, make sure your agni continues to burn bright and strong, and get rid of lymphatic congestion.
- **Adrenal prime:** Swap the Tame the Flame Tea (see page 226) for two cups of tulsi tea per day. You can refer to the section on rasayana (rejuvenation and longevity) for a detailed discussion of tulsi as a superb adaptogenic herb. Because tulsi is energetically slightly warming, I recommend a tulsi-rose blend in the summer to ensure that the body is not overheating.

## *Week 2: Scrub, Mini Fast, Yoga Nidra*

You are now ready to deepen your lymphatic cleansing and start to slowly recalibrate your nervous system.

### Morning Routine

- **Scrub:** Add five to ten minutes of dry-brushing before your (hot-) cold shower routine in the morning. If you are short on time, you can do this in the evening after work and before dinner. Skip the scrub during menstruation, strong Vata or Mover imbalances, or with skin issues such as extreme dryness, eczema, or psoriasis.

### General

- **Mini fast:** One day this week, do a liquid-only fast. I recommend using water fasting for Regenerators or if you have a Kapha imbalance; a juice fast for Transformers or if you have Pitta imbalance; and a soup fast for Movers or if you have Vata imbalance.

  Ideally do this on a day off from work, where you can relax and have time to support your body with additional self-care rituals such as sauna or a massage treatment.

### Evening Ritual

- **Yoga nidra:** To deepen sleep and regenerate your nervous system, twice this week at bedtime do a guided yoga nidra session (twenty minutes). You can find many versions online.

### *Week 3: Lube, Tonify, Gratitude*

Congratulations! You are almost there. In this last week, add a dosha-specific adaptogenic and rejuvenating herb to gently rebuild your physical and nervous system resilience.

#### Morning Routine

- **Lube:** Alternate dry-brushing with self-oil massage (*abhyanga*) in the morning or before bed. In fall and winter, or if you are a Mover type, you can gently warm the oil before doing the massage.

#### General

- **Tonify adrenals:** Start adding an adaptogenic herb such as ashwagandha, rhodiola, or brahmi to your supplement routine, from this week onward, for at least three months.
- **Movers:** Ashwagandha (*Withania somnifera*)—Ayurveda's most famous adaptogen that is superbly grounding, builds resilience, balances stress, and restores vitality. Take one capsule after breakfast and at bedtime with warm water or a half teaspoon of herb powder cooked into (plant-based) milk or water for five minutes.
- **Transformers:** Brahmi (*Bacopa monnieri*)—a revered Ayurvedic herb used for calming the nervous system, improving memory, and enhancing focus. Take one capsule or a half teaspoon of herb powder twice a day with warm water, in between meals.
- **Regenerators:** Rhodiola (*Rhodiola rosea*)—a hardy adaptogenic herb native to Siberia that boosts resilience to stress, enhances energy, and supports mental clarity. Take one capsule twice a day with warm water in between meals.

#### Evening Ritual

- **Gratitude:** Add a gratitude practice. Before falling asleep, make it a habit to recall three beautiful things that happened during the day and connect to the feeling of gratitude in your heart.

## The Summit

Congratulations! You have made your way through all three phases of our Ayurvedic reboot. You have rewired your circadian rhythm, boosted agni, detoxified gut and lymph, and started to recalibrate your mind. By now you have developed a sense of what you need to feel good, energized, and calm. In short, you know how health and balance feel in your body and mind. And you can now better gauge whether a food or lifestyle choice you make is right for you.

After your journey, it is time to assess your imbalances (*vikriti*), gut function (*agni*), and level of toxicity (*ama*) once more. Please redo the three tests that you filled out at the beginning of your journey and compare. If you still have imbalances and toxicity, I recommend redoing the program, possibly this time directly on the Turbo Track or until your tests come out balanced. If you have improved in all three areas, then you are ready to move on to a maintenance program. Here you get to decide which parts of the nine- or eighteen-week journey you want to keep for yourself—for now or for the rest of your life. To help you make a choice, I list below what I consider to be the living Ayurveda 2.0 maintenance essentials.

### *How to Stay at Peak: Your Living Ayurveda 2.0 Maintenance Program*

**Top Three Morning Hacks.** Your morning sets the tone for the day. These are my top three morning hacks that I never skip, no matter how busy the rest of my day is.

1. **Early rise:** Harness the power of early sunlight by getting up before or around sunrise.
2. **Cleanse:** Scrape—get rid of ama on your tongue. Scrub—dry-brush to boost lymphatics, especially in spring; or lube—oil up, especially in fall and winter. Contrast (cold) shower.
3. **Hydrate:** Warm (lemon-honey) water instead of coffee or tea flushes the liver and intestines and rehydrates the body.

Top Three Evening Hacks. Your evening determines how good you feel the next morning, so my advice is at least five days a week, keep it early and light.

1. **Early light dinner:** Close the kitchen by 7 p.m.
2. **Digital detox:** Switch off electronics (or wear blue-light-blocking glasses) by 9 p.m. at the latest.
3. **Early bedtime:** Get to bed no later than 10 p.m. or 11 p.m.

Lifestyle Hacks. Making lunch your biggest meal and dinner light and early will be one of the easiest and most effective ways to enhance your digestive and metabolic power.

- **Twelve to sixteen hours of intermittent fasting:** Close the kitchen by 7 p.m. and reopen for breakfast timed according to your type the next morning.
- **Make lunch the biggest meal:** This sustains you through the Vata or Mover afternoon slump and curbs sugar and coffee cravings.

Food Hacks. Eating right is incredibly simple. If I had to sum up for you in one sentence how to eat to live past age one hundred, I would use the writer Michael Pollan's famous quote: "Eat food, mostly plants, not too much."[2] So instead of getting caught in the latest food craze, stick to this simple wisdom: Eat real, home-cooked, fresh, and whole foods; eat mostly plants with (optionally) small amounts of high-quality animal protein; and do not overeat (remember our *yogi, bhogi, rogi* saying). This simple wisdom sums up explorer and author Dan Buettner's groundbreaking research on the "Blue Zones," regions around the world such as Sardinia (Italy), Ikaria (Greece), or Okinawa (Japan), where the highest concentration of centenarians live and age-related disease incidents are unusually low.

Here are a few of my Ayurvedic food hack additions:

1. **Avoid incompatible food combos.** Especially fruit combined with meals or dairy with meat or fish.

2. **Avoid leftovers.** Cook fresh as much as possible.
3. **Eat seasonal.** Shop at a local farmers market to know what the harvest is.
4. **Use ghee.** Especially in higher-heat cooking.
5. **Use digestive spices.** Spices help to boost digestion and absorption.
6. **Use agni reset teas.** These teas support you at times of need, especially when you eat out or when your digestive strength is low.

Herbal Hacks. At times when you need extra support, these are a few of my favorite Ayurvedic herbs and spices that are unbeatable.

- **Triphala:** An all-rounder for bowel detox, antioxidant support, and cellular rejuvenation.
- **Turmeric:** My number one anti-inflammatory spice.
- **Ashwagandha:** The best adaptogenic support for a strong, muscular body, a resilient and calm nervous system, and deep rejuvenating sleep.

# Part Four

## Living Ayurveda 2.0: Kitchen Secrets

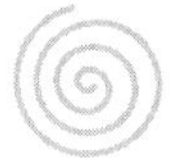

Last but not least, we meet in the kitchen. In this section I invite you to embark on a flavorful journey to discover key recipes that form the foundation of your living Ayurveda 2.0 journey. The recipes are simple, quick, modular, and carefully crafted to support your body on your path toward vitality and well-being. And they are so delicious that you will come back to them repeatedly, even after you have finished your program. From aromatic spice blends to nourishing broths, from vibrant lunch bowls to soothing herbal teas, I promise you that these recipes will become your Ayurvedic kitchen essentials. And they will seduce you into a deeper connection with the delicious healing power of food.

# 9

# The Essentials

## Agni Reset Teas

### Fire Up Tea

This is a great digestive and immune-boosting tea that can be enjoyed by all constitutions in fall and winter, but it should be used with caution by Transformers or in summer. It stimulates circulation, boosts antioxidant levels, and enhances lymphatic flow, all vital to keep you healthy and strong during flu season. In fall, I add a few slices of the Chinese herb astragalus root (*huang qi*) to this tea mixture, for the added immune and qi-tonic benefits.

Makes 2 cups

3–4 slices fresh ginger root
1 tsp goji berries
2 cups water

1. Boil the ginger and goji berries in two cups of water, covered, for 15–20 minutes.
2. Strain and fill into a thermos.
3. Enjoy sip by sip between meals throughout the day.

*Shortcut:* If you are pressed for time, you can finely chop the ginger and add it along with the goji berries directly into a thermos, add boiling water, cover, and let it steep in the thermos for at least 15–20 minutes.

### Tame the Flame Tea

When I studied at Dr. Vasant Lad's Ayurvedic Institute in New Mexico, a pot of this tea was always brewing in our classroom. To this day, drinking a cup brings back many beautiful memories from that time. This is a fantastic tea to enhance digestion and assimilation of nutrients for all seasons and constitutions. It is also considered alkalinizing to the body and a great adjunct for treating urinary tract infections. I usually roast a large batch of the seeds and keep them ready in a jar to make the tea as needed.

Makes 2 cups

1 tsp fennel seeds
1 tsp coriander seeds
1 tsp cumin seeds
2 cups water

1. Dry-roast the seeds in a pan for several minutes, until an aromatic smell develops. You can also roast a larger batch and keep it in a jar.
2. Transfer to a pot and pour boiling water over it. Cover and simmer the decoction for 010–15 minutes, then strain and enjoy with or in between meals.

*Shortcut:* If you are pressed for time, you can add the seeds directly into a thermos, add boiling water, cover, and let it steep in the thermos, for at least 15–20 minutes.

## Agni Reset Spices

### Ayurvedic Ginger Pickle

According to Ayurveda, ginger awakens the taste buds, gets digestive juices flowing, and enhances absorption. This classic Ayurvedic recipe has been used for thousands of years to promote strong digestive power (*agni*). I often call it "Ayurvedic digestive enzymes." Great for Movers and Regenerators, but too heating for Transformers.

Makes 6–8 pickles

¾ inch of fresh ginger root
½ lemon, squeezed
¼ tsp Himalayan pink salt
¼ tsp ground black pepper

1. Peel the ginger and cut it into thin slices. Pour the lemon juice over the ginger.
2. Sprinkle with the salt and black pepper and mix. Allow the ginger to marinate for 1 hour.
3. Eat one slice 10 minutes before a meal to kindle agni.

### Fire Up Spice (Trikatu Churna)

This is Ayurveda's go-to formula for digestive trouble such as low appetite, indigestion, and problems with absorption and assimilation. It is also a great formula for colds and congestion. Fire Up Spice tastes great sautéed in a little ghee or coconut oil and drizzled over soup, beans, or veggies, especially in fall and winter. Be careful not to overuse this in summer or in Transformers since it is extremely pungent.

Serves 70 (½ tsp servings)

¼ cup ground black pepper
¼ cup pippali (Indian long pepper) powder
¼ cup ground ginger

1. Mix the three spice powders and store in a jar.
2. Use in cooking or sprinkle on foods as needed.

*Tip:* For cold, cough, and congestion, mix this powder with enough honey to make a paste, and lick a ½ teaspoon every 4 hours.

### Tame the Flame Spice (Hingvasthak Churna)

This is Ayurveda's go-to formula for digestive trouble such as gas and bloating, cramping, and malabsorption. It tastes great, too, sautéed in a little ghee or coconut oil and drizzled over soup, beans, or veggies. I fill a small shaker with the spice mix and take it with me when I eat out. The main star of the formula is asafetida or hing, a pungent resin that is a superb digestive and an essential spice for Mover constitutions.

SERVES 140 (½ TSP SERVINGS)

¼ cup cumin seeds
¼ cup ajwain seeds
¼ cup ground asafetida/hing
½ tsp ghee or coconut oil
¼ cup black peppercorns
¼ cup ground ginger
¼ cup pippali (Indian long pepper) powder
1 tbsp Indian black salt (or, alternatively, Himalayan pink salt)

1. Dry-roast the cumin and ajwain seeds in a small pan for a few minutes. Be careful not to burn.
2. In a separate pan, roast the asafetida/hing in the ghee or coconut oil for 1 minute, until it develops an aromatic smell and the color slightly darkens.
3. When the seeds are cooled, grind them along with the black peppercorns in a coffee grinder.
4. Mix the ground seeds with the ground ginger, pippali powder, roasted ground asafetida/hing, and salt and store in a jar.
5. Sprinkle on foods as needed or take ¼ teaspoon under the tongue after meals for better absorption.

## HAPPY BELLY SPICE

You cannot miss the bowl of vibrantly green seeds at the entrance of almost any Indian restaurant, where they are offered as a breath freshener after a spicy or garlicky meal. In addition to neutralizing bad breath, fennel seeds are also a fantastic digestive remedy for all constitutions, especially if you tend to get acidity, bloating, or gas after meals. I always have a small jar in my purse when I eat out as a quick and simple digestive soother.

SERVES 48 (½ TSP SERVINGS)

1 cup fennel seeds

1. Dry-roast the fennel seeds in a pan for 3–4 minutes or until a fragrant smell develops and the seeds turn lightly golden.
2. Store in an airtight container and chew ½ teaspoon of seeds after meals to counter gas and bloating.

*Note:* If I want to be fancy, I add 3 tablespoons coconut flakes and ½ teaspoon freshly ground cardamom to the fennel seeds when roasting. This renders the mix sweet and nutty and curbs any sweet cravings after a meal.

# 10

## Liquid Tonics

### Morning Lemon Water

INSTEAD of starting the day with coffee or tea, which drains kidney energy and stresses the adrenals, Ayurveda recommends drinking a mix of lemon, honey, and water to help flush out toxins, stimulate the bowels, and hydrate the body. Both honey and lemon help to eliminate excess Kapha or mucous from the body. In summer, or for Transformer types, omit the honey and switch to lime, which is cooling. Also, if you are intermittent fasting, omit the honey or drink this 30 minutes before your first meal.

SERVES 2

2 cups warm water
½–1 lemon, juiced (depending on how tart you like it)
2 tsp honey (optional)

1. Bring the water to boil, then let it cool to about 45°C or mix with a little cold water. (Remember, according to the classical texts, honey becomes toxic when heated.)
2. Add the lemon juice and honey (optional) and drink on an empty stomach in the mornings.

### Deep-Sleep Tonic

Poppy-seed milk is a popular and effective sleep remedy and staple in many Indian grandmas' households. Combining nutmeg with poppy seeds is especially effective as both herbs by themselves are powerful sedatives but each have different action times. Nutmeg needs several hours before its maximum sedative effect kicks in, so it is a suitable remedy for people who fall asleep easily but wake up in the middle of the night. Poppy seeds, on the contrary, are fast-acting but the action wears off after a few hours, so they're great if you have trouble falling asleep. By combining the two, you get the benefits of both worlds and a superb, sustained sleep combo. It works especially well for Movers' hypernervous system.

SERVES 1

1 tsp poppy seeds

1 cup milk of choice (cow, goat, or plant-based milks such as almond, oat, or hemp)

¼ cup water

¼ tsp freshly grated nutmeg

1 tsp sweetener, such as coconut sugar or maple syrup (optional)

1. Dry-roast the poppy seeds in a pan for a few minutes until the color slightly darkens and a fragrant aroma develops. Let cool and grind them into a paste using a mortar and pestle. (If needed, add 1–2 tablespoons of water while grinding to make aju thick paste.)
2. Return the poppy seed paste to the pan and add the milk, water, and nutmeg. Let the mixture come to a boil, then turn the heat to low and let it simmer for 5–10 minutes, stirring continuously.
3. Turn off the heat and pour into a mug. If desired, add 1 teaspoon of sweetener (or to taste) and mix well.

*Upgrade:* Add ½ teaspoon ashwagandha powder to this mix when boiling the milk. It gives an extra layer of adaptogenic and sleep support.

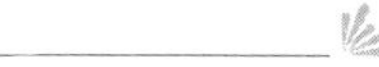

## AYURVEDIC PROTEIN POWER SHAKE

This shake is a great light breakfast or post-workout energy boost, suitable for Movers and Transformers. Soothing, nourishing, and grounding, it makes an ideal snack for people on the go. You can adjust the thickness to your liking by adding more water. The cardamom helps digestion and adds a lovely flavor. Optional ashwagandha and collagen add a layer of muscle and connective-tissue support that I love in this shake.

Serves 2

½ cup raw almonds
3 dates
4 cups filtered water, divided
¼ tsp ground cardamom
½ tsp ashwagandha root powder (optional)
1 tbsp collagen powder (optional)

1. Soak the almonds and dates separately, in 1 cup filtered water, overnight. Make sure to discard all the date pits, otherwise they will ruin your blender.
2. Transfer almonds to a blender, add 2 cups water, and blend on high speed for 1 minute. Strain almond milk using a nut milk bag or cheesecloth.
3. Add the strained milk along with the soaked dates, cardamom, ashwagandha (optional), and collagen (optional), and blend again until smooth.
4. Enjoy at room temperature or lightly warmed.

*Note:* The remaining almond pulp can be used in your porridge for breakfast or as a thickener in soups. I usually dry it in the oven at the lowest setting, then grind it into flour and use it in baking.

### Probiotic Beet Kvass

Ever since I made my first batch of kvass, I have been in love with this pink effervescent beverage that is slightly sour and a kick-ass probiotic digestive aid. I usually have a glass with lunch or dinner during fall and winter. Beet kvass is balancing to Movers and Regenerators, but as a ferment, it can be too heating for Transformers and during the summer months.

Makes about 8 cups

3 large beets, peeled and chopped into quarters
1 tsp Himalayan pink salt
¼ cup fresh whey or the contents of a probiotic capsule, as a probiotic-rich starter culture (optional)
4 cups filtered water

1. Place the beets in a jar, sprinkle with the salt, add the whey (or the contents of a probiotic capsule), then add the water. The whey helps to speed up the fermentation but can also be omitted.
2. Cover the jar and allow the kvass to ferment at room temperature for 3 days, depending on the temperature in your kitchen.
3. Strain the beets from the kvass and reserve them, as well as a ½ cup of the liquid, for culturing your next batch. The beets should be good for one or two more batches and after can be discarded.
4. Kvass should be stored in the refrigerator (where it usually keeps for 3 weeks) and can be enjoyed with meals as a digestive and probiotic tonic.

### How to Obtain Whey

You can get probiotic-rich whey easily by taking a spoon of the semi-opaque liquid that naturally separates from your yogurt in its container. If there is none, then strain your yogurt for half an hour using a cheese cloth. The liquid that drains out is whey.

# 11

## Gut-Healing Foods

### Turmeric Ghee

Ghee, or clarified butter, is made by cooking unsalted (sour cream) butter at low heat for an extended period, until the milk solids or proteins sink to the bottom of the pot. Once the proteins are discarded, what remains is pure butter oil, which Ayurveda also calls "liquid gold" due to its amazing medicinal properties. Sweet, cooling, and light, ghee is considered one of the most rejuvenating, antiaging, and nourishing foods. Ghee balances all three doshas, rejuvenates all seven tissues, nourishes, and improves digestion, absorption, and assimilation. This is the reason that in Ayurvedic medicine, many herbal preparations are cooked into or administered with ghee. Ghee is also highly heat-stable and thus a great general oil for higher-heat cooking.

Makes about 28 ounces

2 pounds unsalted, organic, cultured (sour cream) butter
1 tbsp ground turmeric
8 whole black peppercorns or pippali (Indian long pepper) (optional)

1. Melt the butter over low to medium heat in a large pot, then continue simmering it for at least 1 hour. Do not touch or stir. When the milk solids start settling to the bottom of the pan and turn golden, the surface starts to clear, and the butter looks more like oil, scoop off any remaining solids that float on top.
2. Turn off the heat, add the ground turmeric (don't stir), and let the ghee sit for another 20 minutes. Then pour the ghee through a cheesecloth into clean or sterilized glass jars. Let the ghee cool to room temperature before you cover the jars because otherwise the condensation water will spoil the ghee.

*Note:* Because all the milk proteins are removed, ghee has an indefinite shelf life. In fact, the older the ghee, the more medicinal it becomes. Ghee does not need to be refrigerated—actually, it never should be. When ghee turns solid in the fridge, its properties change and the cold quality gets "imprinted" into the ghee, which greatly diminishes its digestion-enhancing and lubricating power.

### Gut-Healing Marrow Bone (or Chicken) Broth

Bone broth is enjoying a rising popularity as a medicinal, gut-healing drink. It is rich in collagen and gelatin, both important not only for bone, tendon, and skin health but also for rebuilding the lining of the digestive tract. Collagen is rich in the amino acids glycine and proline, and plays a crucial role in providing structural support, strength, and elasticity to the tissues in the body. Collagen is especially helpful in rebuilding the lining of the gut in conditions such as leaky gut, inflammatory bowel diseases, and autoimmune conditions. Bone broth is considered tri-doshic, but Transformers and Regenerators may want to scoop off any excess fat.

Makes 45 fl oz broth

5–6 marrow bones, with some meat and fat still on the bone, or one whole chicken, with meat removed and bones chopped (In Turkey, we generally use collagen-rich lamb feet.)

68 fl oz filtered water

½ tsp baking soda (optional)

1½ cups vegetable scraps (beet tops; onion, potato, celery, or carrot peels and tops; broccoli stems; leafy green stalks, etc.); if scraps are not available, use ½ onion, 1 carrot, 1 potato, and 1–2 slices celery root

6 shitake mushrooms

3 tbsp apple cider vinegar

2 cloves garlic, bruised with the back of a knife (this potentizes allicin content and flavor of the garlic)

2 bay leaves

8 whole black peppercorns

4 slices fresh ginger rhizome

1 tsp ground turmeric

1 tbsp goji berries

1 strip kombu

1. Place the marrow bones (or lamb feet) in a pot and cover with cold water. Add the baking soda (optional), turn on the heat, and bring to a boil. After boiling for about 5 minutes, discard the water and rinse the bones. This helps remove any impurities from the bones. If you have an organic chicken, this step is not necessary.
2. Place the bones back in the pot, fill new with 68 fl oz filtered water, and add the vegetables, mushrooms, vinegar, garlic, bay leaves, black peppercorns, ginger slices, turmeric, goji berries, and kombu.
3. Bring to a boil. Once the water boils, turn down the heat a little and cook for at least 12 hours, but better up to 24 hours. You may need to add more water during this long cooking process. Always add boiling water to not disturb or halt the cooking.
4. When the broth is ready, and the water content approximately reduced to two-thirds, strain out the solids and pour the broth into jars. Once cooled, refrigerate until the top fat layer consolidates. Unless you need fat, extra calories, and lubrication (Movers), discard (at least part of) this (highly saturated) fat layer.
5. You can keep the broth in the fridge for up to 3 days before it starts turning sour. Or you can freeze it in small jars for convenient later use. While Ayurveda is not a big fan of using frozen foods because nutrition diminishes and the cold quality gets imprinted into the food, thus interfering with agni, one exception I make is broth since it is impossible to make daily but is such a vital and nourishing base for many of my meals.

*Note:* When making bone broth, it is vital to cook the bones for an extended time (at least 12 hours) at minimal heat, and always use an additional acidic medium such as lemon or apple cider vinegar to facilitate the release of minerals and collagen from the bones.

### Gut-Healing Vegan Miso Broth

This broth is a very simple recipe to prepare and a great vegan alternative to the gut-healing bone broth. Garlic and thyme are antibacterial and support a healthy gut lining; the coconut oil and turmeric ease inflammation; and miso adds vital beneficial bacteria and supports bowel flora.

MAKES 45 FL OZ OF BROTH

- 1 tbsp organic, extra-virgin coconut oil
- 4 cups vegetable scraps (beet tops; onion, potato, celery, or carrot peels and tops; broccoli stems; leafy green stalks, etc.); if scraps are not available, use ½ onion, 2 carrots, 1 potato, and 1–2 slices celery root
- 6 shitake mushrooms (fresh or dried)
- ½-inch piece ginger root, sliced
- 2 cloves garlic, bruised with the back of a knife (this potentizes allicin content and flavor of the garlic)
- 8 whole black peppercorns
- 1 tsp turmeric
- 1 tsp dried or fresh thyme
- 52 fl oz filtered water
- 1 strip kombu
- 3 tbsp sweet mild shiro (white) miso paste

1. Gently heat the coconut oil in a pot and add the vegetable scraps, mushrooms, ginger, garlic, black peppercorns, turmeric, and thyme. Sauté for 2–3 minutes, then add the water and kombu strip and cover with a lid.
2. Bring the mixture to a boil, then turn down the heat and leave the broth to a simmer for 1 hour.
3. Turn off the heat and let it cool to warm. Strain well and discard the solids.
4. Whisk in the miso paste and drink 1 cup right away. Store the rest for up to 3 days in the fridge, or you can freeze it in small jars for convenient later use.

### TONIC KITCHARI

Kitchari is a simple, satisfying one-pot meal that is delicious, nourishing, and easy to digest. In Ayurveda, it is often the food of choice during periods of detoxification (*panchakarma*) or when digestion is low, and it is balancing to all three constitutions. Soaking the mung dal overnight reduces cooking time and releases enzyme-inhibitors, such as phytic acid, contained in all beans, grains, nuts, and seeds, which can create digestive difficulty and block the absorption of minerals.

SERVES 4

½ tsp coriander seeds
1 tsp cumin seeds
2 tbsp ghee
½ tsp black mustard seeds
½ onion, chopped
1 tsp fresh ginger root, grated
A few pinches asafetida/hing (optional)
½ tsp ground turmeric
1 cup basmati rice, washed and soaked for 30 minutes
½ cup mung dal (split mung beans), soaked overnight
4 cups water (you can increase it up to 6 cups if you want a creamier or soupier version)
½ tsp Himalayan pink salt
1 bay leaf
1 cinnamon stick
1 cup chopped veggies (either single or mixed such as spinach, chard, zucchini, carrots, etc.)
Ground black pepper, to taste

1. Dry-roast the coriander and cumin seeds for 1–2 minutes, let cool, and grind them with a coffee grinder or mortar and pestle. (If you have powder, omit this step, and use the same amount as the seeds.)
2. Heat the ghee in a pot and add the mustard seeds. When they start to splutter, add the onion and sauté for 5 minutes. Add the ginger, asafetida/hing, turmeric, and dry-roasted coriander and cumin powders and sauté for 1 minute. Add the soaked basmati rice and mung dal and sauté for 1 minute.
3. Add the water, salt, bay leaf, cinnamon stick, and vegetables, bring to a boil, then simmer on low heat for 20 minutes, until all the water is absorbed and the kitchari has a soft and creamy consistency.
4. Remove the cinnamon stick and bay leaf, and season to taste with additional salt and ground black pepper. Serve with toppings of your choice. Here are a few ideas:

- Chopped fresh herbs such as dill (Movers), cilantro (Transformers), or parsley (Regenerators)
- Dollop of ghee (Movers, Transformers)
- Squeeze of lemon (Movers, Regenerators)
- Chili flakes (Regenerators)
- Toasted coconut flakes (Transformers)

*Note:* If you are pressed for time, overwhelmed or just a little lazy ☺, you can also cook the mung dal, basmati rice, and vegetables, along with some salt, in one pot for 20 minutes. In the meantime, heat 2 tablespoons of ghee in a separate pan, add 1 or 2 teaspoons of curry powder, sauté for 1 minute at low heat, then add it to the cooked kitchari at the end.

# 12

## Easy Breakfasts

### Freestyle Morning Porridge

Ayurveda loves to start the day with a light, warm, and easy-to-digest meal that breaks your fast from overnight without overburdening agni. But if you are bored of oatmeal with raisins, here is an invitation to build your own, ever-changing breakfast bowl, tailor-made to your individual needs and tastes. If sweet is not your thing, you can cook your porridge in a little ghee with spices such as ginger, cumin, and coriander, and top it with roasted seeds, a poached egg or tempeh, fresh herbs (e.g., parsley, dill, or cilantro), and a squeeze of lemon. The concept is simple.

Serves 1

1. Base and spices: Dry-roast your grains or flakes of choice (¼–½ cup per serving) with ¼ teaspoon spices in a small pot for 2–3 minutes.
2. Liquid: Add ½–1 cup water and/or milk of choice. Cover, bring to boil, then simmer for 10 minutes (flakes) or 20 minutes (whole grains), or until the porridge is thick and creamy. At this stage, if you like, you can also add your
   - Add-ons: chopped dried fruits (dates, goji berries, figs, etc.)
   - Superfoods: ½ teaspoon maca or ashwagandha, or 1 teaspoon raw cacao nibs or chia seeds
3. Topping: Dry-roast 1 tablespoon chopped nuts and/or seeds for your topping.
4. Sweetener: Stir in sweetener, nut butter, or tahini (optional).
5. Serve topped with roasted nuts and an additional sprinkle of spices.

*Note:* If you want to use fresh fruit, keep in mind that combining fresh fruit with other foods is not optimal food combining, according to

Ayurveda. If you want to add fruit to your morning bowl, always use only a small amount of cooked (!) fruit as a condiment, such as a few slices of ghee-fried caramelized banana or cooked apple.

| | Movers | Transformers | Regenerators |
|---|---|---|---|
| Base | Oats, quinoa, amaranth (whole or flakes); ground tigernut | Oats, quinoa, millet, amaranth (whole or flakes) | Millet, buckwheat, amaranth (whole or flakes); ground cornmeal (polenta) |
| Liquids | Water, almond milk, hemp milk, oat milk | Water, rice milk, oat milk, coconut milk | Water, rice milk |
| Add-Ons (dried) | Dates, figs, apricots, raisins, berries | Dates, figs, apricots, raisins, berries | Berries, raisins |
| Spices | Cinnamon, cardamom, ginger, saffron, vanilla, fresh orange or lemon zest | Cardamom, turmeric, saffron, vanilla | Cinnamon, cardamom, ginger, turmeric, saffron, vanilla, fresh orange or lemon zest |
| Superfoods | Maca, ashwagandha, raw cacao nibs, chia seeds, goji berries | Maca, chia seeds, raw cacao nibs, goji berries | Ashwagandha, raw cacao nibs, chia seeds, goji berries |
| Toppings | 1. Roasted nuts and seeds (almonds, walnuts, hemp, sesame; coconut chips) | 1. Roasted seeds (sunflower, pumpkin, hemp; coconut chips) | 1. Roasted seeds (sunflower, pumpkin, hempseeds) |

| | Movers | Transformers | Regenerators |
|---|---|---|---|
| Toppings (continued) | 2. Almond butter or tahini<br>3. Small amount of cooked fruit (bananas, pears, figs, peaches, persimmons) | 2. Small amount of cooked fruit (peaches, apricots, pomegranate, apple, pear) | 2. Small amount of cooked fruit (berries, pomegranate, apple, pear) |
| Sweeteners | Date syrup, molasses, coconut sugar | Date or maple syrup, coconut sugar | None, or a small amount of honey (be careful not to heat) |

Need more inspiration? Here are some of my favorite go-tos:

### Mover Porridge

Oat-quinoa porridge for protein power, cooked with water and almond milk, ashwagandha (optional), chopped dates, and cinnamon; and topped with caramelized banana slices, tahini, and roasted almonds.

### Transformer Porridge

Millet porridge for alkalinity, cooked with water and coconut milk, cacao nibs, and cardamom; and topped with a few slices of vanilla-poached peaches and roasted hempseeds.

### Regenerator Porridge

Polenta porridge for lightness, cooked with water and rice milk, saffron, ginger, and fresh orange zest; and topped with cooked berries and chia seeds.

### All-Rounder Ayurvedic Granola

This homemade tri-doshic granola is lovely served on top of creamy fresh (coconut) yogurt or kefir, drizzled with some additional maple syrup for added sweetness if desired. Alternatively, it can be served as a breakfast cereal with warm (rice, almond, or coconut) milk. I like to have some on hand for mornings when I am short on time.

SERVES 10

3 cups mixed whole-grain flakes (oats, amaranth, quinoa, millet, buckwheat)
A pinch Himalayan pink salt
3 tbsp ghee or coconut oil
½ cup maple or date syrup, or coconut sugar
1 tbsp freshly grated orange peel (from organic, unsprayed oranges)
1 tbsp ashwagandha or maca powder (optional)
½ tsp freshly ground cardamom
1 tsp ground cinnamon
2 tbsp tahini
¼ cup raw sunflower seeds
¼ cup pumpkin seeds
½ cup almonds, chopped, and coconut flakes
½ cup shelled unsalted pistachios (optional)
½ cup dried cherries (or any dried berry of your choice, such as cranberries, raisins, or blueberries)

1. Preheat the oven to 150°C and line a baking sheet with parchment paper.
2. Mix the whole-grain flakes and salt in a bowl. Melt the ghee or coconut oil with the sweetener, orange peel, (optional) ashwagandha or maca, cardamom, and cinnamon in a saucepan over medium heat. Stir to combine, add the tahini, then pour over the whole-grain flake mixture and mix thoroughly using a spatula or your hands.
3. Spread the granola mixture evenly onto the parchment paper–lined baking sheet and bake for at least 20 minutes. Stir, and be careful not to burn.
4. Add the seeds, coconut, almonds, and pistachios. Bake for another 15 minutes, stirring frequently. Make sure the nuts don't burn.
5. Remove from the oven, let cool, then add the dried cherries or berries. Store in an airtight container.
6. Serve with homemade (coconut) yogurt or kefir or some warm (rice, almond, or coconut) milk.

## Protein Power Green Shakshuka

This green shakshuka—my version of the Israeli egg dish cooked in a spicy tomato sauce—is a great way to use up all the vegetables you have in your refrigerator. I generally use a mix of sturdy greens (kale, collard greens, spinach) and leeks. It is a great alternative for those who love shakshuka but are avoiding nightshade vegetables such as tomatoes or peppers.

Serves 4

- 2 tbsp ghee or coconut oil
- ½ onion, chopped
- ¼ tsp asafetida/hing
- ¼ tsp ground turmeric
- ½ tsp ground cumin
- ½ tsp smoked Spanish paprika (optional)
- ½ bunch kale, stems removed
- ½ bunch collard greens and/or spinach
- ½ stalk leek, white or light green parts, chopped finely
- ¼–½ cup water
- 1 cup fresh herbs (parsley, dill, cilantro, or basil), chopped
- 4 large eggs (or mashed tofu)
- Himalayan pink salt, to taste
- Ground black pepper, to taste
- Black cumin seeds, for topping (optional)
- Sumac, for topping (optional)
- Red pepper (chili) flakes, for topping (optional)

1. Heat the ghee in a cast-iron pan. Add the chopped onion and cook for a few minutes, until the onion has softened. Add the asafetida/hing, turmeric, cumin, and smoked Spanish paprika and sauté 1 minute, then add the sturdy greens (kale, collard greens, spinach, etc.) and leeks and cook until they start to wilt, 3 to 4 minutes. Add ¼–½ cup water and continue cooking for another minute, then add the more delicate chopped herbs. Cook for 1 to 2 minutes.
2. Using a wooden spoon or spatula, create four wells inside the bed of greens. Crack an egg into each well and cover the pan. The eggs will steam-cook; they're ready when the whites are no longer translucent but the yolks are still liquid.
3. Season with salt and black pepper to taste. You can also sprinkle some black cumin seeds, sumac, and/or red pepper flakes on top. Serve with toasted bread of your choice or a side of quinoa.

# 13

## Simple Meals

### Freestyle Lunch Bowl

I love bowl meals. They are super-easy to assemble and can be varied according to what you have in the fridge. Basically there are four layers that can produce endless variations: a grain base or colorful starchy vegetables; greens and other non-starchy vegetables; a protein (plant-based or animal); and a sauce that brings it all together. Depending on the season and the mood you are in, you can vary each of the components. The concept is similar to our breakfast porridge variations from earlier.

Serves 1

1. Base: Cook ¼–½ cup grain of choice in ½–1 cup water *and/or* toss your starchy root vegetables (beets, pumpkin, sweet potatoes, carrots) with a heat-stable oil such as ghee or coconut oil and spices of choice and roast in the oven at 180°C for 20 minutes.
2. Greens: Stir-fry the non-starchy veggies (zucchini, pepper, beans, broccoli, chard, etc.) with optional spices (cumin, smoked Spanish paprika, chili) in a little ghee or coconut oil. If you use leafy salad greens such as arugula or baby spinach, no need to cook.
3. Protein: Grill fish, or chicken, *or* cook your beans or lentils, *or* pan-fry your tempeh or eggs.
4. Dressing: Combine fat (e.g., olive oil, hemp oil, flax oil, tahini), acid (e.g., lemon, vinegar, pomegranate molasses), spice (e.g., mustard, cumin), and sweet (e.g., maple syrup, honey). Adjust the taste by adding Himalayan pink salt and ground black pepper.
5. Topping: Roasted nuts and seeds, chopped dried fruit (e.g., figs, cranberries), seaweed flakes, nutritional yeast, black cumin seeds.

| | Movers | Transformers | Regenerators |
|---|---|---|---|
| Hearty Base | Cooked grains (basmati, jasmine, red or wild rice; amaranth; quinoa; couscous); rice noodles<br><br>*and/or*<br><br>Roasted starchy root veggies (beets, carrots, sweet potatoes, pumpkin) | Cooked grains (basmati, jasmine, red or wild rice; quinoa, millet, buckwheat); soba noodles<br><br>*and/or*<br><br>Roasted starchy root veggies (sweet potatoes, squashes, pumpkin) | Omit grains or use less (basmati or wild rice; millet, buckwheat, polenta)<br><br>*or*<br><br>Small amount of roasted starchy root veggies (beets, carrots, celery root, sunchokes) |
| Colorful Veggies | Small amount of steamed or roasted non-starchy veggies (leeks, zucchini, snow peas, mushrooms, green beans, fennel)<br><br>Small amount of stir-fried or lightly steamed greens (spinach, chard) or fresh herbs (arugula, basil, dill) | Steamed or roasted non-starchy veggies (cauliflower, broccoli, cabbage, leeks, snow peas, green beans, fennel, mushrooms, corn)<br><br>Plenty of stir-fried, lightly steamed, or raw greens (spinach, kale, chard, arugula, mint, cilantro, parsley, dill) | Plenty of steamed or roasted non-starchy veggies (cauliflower, broccoli, cabbage, leeks, snow peas, green beans, fennel, mushrooms, corn)<br><br>Plenty of stir-fried, lightly steamed, or raw greens (spinach, kale, chard, arugula, mint, cilantro, parsley, dill) |
| Plant Protein | Prefer small legumes (mung beans, lentils), tempeh | All legumes (chickpeas, fava, mung beans, lentils), tempeh | All legumes (chickpeas, fava, mung beans, lentils), tempeh |

| | Movers | Transformers | Regenerators |
|---|---|---|---|
| or Animal Protein | Oily fish such as wild-caught salmon, mackerel, or sardines; grilled organic chicken thighs; eggs; fresh goat cheese or mozzarella | Trout or other white fish; grilled organic chicken breast; eggs; fresh goat cheese or mozzarella | Not necessary. If desired, add small amounts of grilled organic chicken breast or white fish; eggs; fresh goat cheese |
| Dressing | 1. Healthy fats (olive, hempseed, or pumpkin seed oil); tahini, almond butter<br>2. Acid (lemon, lime, apple cider vinegar, balsamic vinegar, pomegranate molasses)<br>3. Sweet (maple, date, or coconut syrup)<br>4. Kick (ginger, cumin, sweet mustard) | 1. Healthy fats (olive, hempseed, flax, or avocado oil)<br>2. Acid (lime, apple cider vinegar, pomegranate molasses)<br>3. Sweet (maple, date, or coconut syrup)<br>4. Kick (coriander, cumin, turmeric, dried mint) | 1. Healthy fats (olive, hempseed, flaxseed, or pumpkin seed oil)<br>2. Acid (lemon, lime, apple cider vinegar, balsamic vinegar, pomegranate molasses)<br>3. Sweet (omit, or use honey)<br>4. Kick (ginger, cumin, mustard, chili, black pepper) |
| Topping | Roasted nuts and seeds; dried dates, figs, apricots; seaweed flakes; nutritional yeast; black cumin seeds | Roasted seeds; raisins or dried berries; seaweed flakes; nutritional yeast | Roasted seeds; seaweed flakes; dried (cran)berries; nutritional yeast; black cumin seeds |

Need more inspiration? Here are my favorite lunch bowls.

### Mover Bowl

Basmati rice with mixed roasted root vegetables, served in a bowl alongside cooked warm red lentil dal and stir-fried spinach and chard. I like to top this with a tahini dressing and fresh herbs, chopped dates, nuts and seeds.

Makes 5 oz or 3–4 servings

#### Tahini-Lemon-Ginger Dressing

½ inch ginger root, grated
¼ cup tahini
¼ cup water
½ lemon, juiced
1 tsp date or coconut syrup
Himalayan pink salt
Ground black pepper

*Note:* The tahini dressing stores well for 3 to 4 days in the refrigerator.

### Transformer Bowl

Quinoa with lightly stir-fried zucchini, corn, and green beans, arranged in your bowl as a base topped with chickpeas and lots of raw greens (arugula, mint, cilantro, dill). I serve this topped with ¼–½ cup creamy avocado dressing and goji berries.

Makes 6 oz or 4 servings

#### Creamy Avocado Dressing

½ avocado
1 cup fresh herbs (parsley, coriander, dill, mint), finely chopped
¼–½ cup water
2 tbsp lemon or lime juice
1 tbsp olive oil
1 tbsp date or maple syrup
Himalayan pink salt
Ground black pepper

*Note:* The avocado dressing keeps well for 1 to 2 days in the refrigerator.

### Regenerator Bowl

Buckwheat with lightly stir-fried green asparagus, broccoli, and leeks, beluga lentils and plenty of fresh herbs and greens (arugula, parsley, etc.). I sprinkle cranberries or fresh pomegranate seeds on top and drizzle 1 or 2 tablespoons of spicy parsley chimichurri over the bowl.

Makes 4 oz or 4 servings

#### Parsley Chimichurri

2 cups flat parsley, finely chopped
½ cup fresh mint leaves, finely chopped
2 cloves garlic, roasted and crushed
1 small shallot, finely chopped
2 tsp dried oregano
½ tsp red pepper flakes
2 tbsp red wine vinegar
¼ tsp Himalayan pink salt
¼ tsp ground black pepper
⅓ cup extra-virgin olive oil

*Note:* The chimichurri keeps for at least 1 week in the refrigerator.

## Sup(P)Er Soups

### Carrot-Ginger Soup

There is nothing like a bowl of sunshine on a cold, windy autumn day. The color of this soup is striking—a bright and deep yellow orange. For me, carrot soup means comfort food. It is sweet, with a kick from the ginger, and creamy from the coconut milk.

Serves 4

2 tbsp ghee or coconut oil
½ onion, chopped
1 lb carrots, peeled and cubed
1 tbsp fresh ginger root, grated
1 cinnamon stick
½ tsp ground turmeric
½ tsp Himalayan pink salt
5–6 cups water (or bone, chicken, or veggie broth)
½ cup full-fat coconut milk (optional)
½ cup fresh parsley, chopped
Freshly ground black pepper, to taste

1. Heat the ghee or coconut oil over medium-high heat in a medium pot. Add the onions, carrots, and ginger and sauté for a few minutes.
2. Add the cinnamon stick and turmeric, and sauté for another minute, then add the salt and water or broth.
3. Bring to boil, turn down heat, cover, and simmer for 20 minutes. Remove the cinnamon stick. For extra creaminess, add the coconut milk.
4. Puree the soup with a hand blender, adjust the seasoning to taste, and add more water to adjust consistency.
5. Serve with the chopped parsley and freshly ground black pepper.

### Beet Bortsch

Beet bortsch is an Eastern European staple. It is said that you can find as many variations of it as there are Russian grandmas. I enjoy this gorgeous, deep-purple soup warm in fall and winter and at room temperature in spring or late summer. If I have the time, I roast the beets whole in the oven before using them to bring out their sweet, deep, caramelized flavor.

Serves 4

1 tbsp ghee or coconut oil
½ onion, chopped
A pinch asafetida/hing
½ tsp ground turmeric
2 carrots, peeled (if not organic) and sliced
3 medium beets, washed, peeled, and cut into chunks
5–6 cups water (or bone, chicken, or veggie broth)
2 bay leaves
1 tbsp goji berries
½ tsp Himalayan pink salt, to taste
Ground black pepper, to taste
Splash apple cider vinegar, to taste

#### To Serve

¼ cup parsley or chives, chopped
4 tbsp strained (goat or coconut) yogurt (optional)

1. Wash and peel the beets, and coarsely chop into chunks. Slice the carrots and chop the parsley and onion.
2. Heat the ghee over medium-high heat in a medium pot. Add the onion and asafetida/hing and sauté for one or two minutes, then add the turmeric, carrots, and beets, and sauté for another minute. Add the broth, bay leaves, goji berries, salt, and black pepper.
3. Bring to a boil, cover, and simmer at low heat for 15 minutes if you pre-roasted your beets, or 30 minutes if you added them in raw form.
4. Remove the bay leaves and puree the soup with a hand blender to a consistency of your liking. Some people prefer their bortsch chunky. I like mine smooth and silky.
5. If needed, add more salt and freshly ground black pepper, and a splash of apple cider vinegar to taste. Serve the bortsch topped with the chopped parsley or chives and dollop of yogurt (optional).

### Green Detox Soup

This is a great detoxifying and blood-cleansing soup that is vibrantly green and tastes amazing. It is best enjoyed in the spring, when nettles are tender and fresh, or throughout the year using a half cup dried nettles alongside fresh greens such as spinach or chard. Movers can enjoy this soup in moderation, perhaps best made with a more nourishing meat broth and additional ghee, and Transformers should omit the smoked paprika or chili.

Serves 4

1 bunch fresh nettles (or ½ cup dried nettles, reconstituted in ½ cup boiling water, alongside one bunch of fresh spinach or chard)

1 tbsp ghee or coconut oil

½ onion, chopped

A pinch asafetida/hing

½ tsp ground turmeric

¼ tsp Spanish smoked paprika and/or chili powder (optional)

5 cups water (or bone, chicken, or veggie broth)

½ tsp Himalayan pink salt

Ground black pepper, to taste

1. Wash the nettles and separate leaves. (You might have to do this with gloves since some varieties can sting.)
2. Heat the ghee or coconut oil over medium-high heat in a medium-sized pot. Add the onion and a pinch of asafetida/hing, and sauté for 1 to 2 minutes, then add the turmeric and smoked paprika or chili (optional), as well as the greens. Sauté for another minute, then add the water or broth and salt.
3. Bring to a boil and then simmer at low heat, covered, for 5 minutes.
4. Turn off the heat and puree the soup with a hand blender until smooth. Add additional salt and freshly ground black pepper to taste.

## Lemony Broccoli Soup

Most people hate broccoli. I think it is a vastly underrated vegetable, and I especially love this soup. While most broccoli soups are made with milk and cream, which is heavy on digestion, this soup is light and bright with the lemon and just a hint of sharp from Parmesan or nutritional yeast, if you like. Make sure to not overcook the broccoli to preserve maximum nutrition.

Serves 4

1 tbsp ghee or coconut oil
1 clove garlic, minced
A pinch asafetida/hing
½ tsp ground turmeric
1 lb broccoli florets, trimmed and cut if needed
½ tsp Himalayan pink salt
Ground black pepper, to taste
5–6 cups water (or bone, chicken, or vegetable broth)
½ organic lemon, juiced and zested

**To Serve**

1 tbsp grated Parmesan or 1 tbsp vegan nutritional yeast (optional)
Crusty sourdough bread

1. In a medium-sized pot, heat the ghee over medium-high heat. When hot, add the garlic and asafetida and sauté, stirring frequently. After a minute or two, when the garlic starts to soften

and turn golden, add the turmeric as well as the broccoli florets. Season with salt and pepper, and stir well.

2. Add the broth, bring to a boil, then reduce the heat to low and simmer, covered, for 10 minutes, until the broccoli is soft but still vibrantly green.
3. Blend the soup with a hand blender, stir in the lemon juice and zest. Taste and adjust the seasoning.
4. Serve hot, sprinkled with the Parmesan or nutritional yeast, and with a slice of crusty sourdough bread.

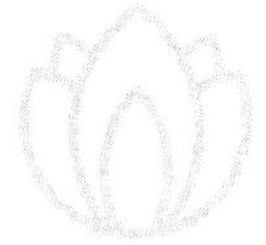

# Glossary

***agni.*** The digestive fire that transforms food into nutrients and energy. A strong agni is essential for good health and efficient metabolism. A weak agni can lead to digestive issues and the accumulation of ama.

***ahara.*** A term meaning "nutrition and diet"; a central concept in Ayurveda. A balanced diet tailored to one's individual constitution is vital for maintaining health and balance. The right food choices can help prevent and even heal disease.

***ama.*** Toxic residues and undigested substances that accumulate in the body and can cause illness. These endotoxins are produced by weak digestion and low agni. The elimination of ama is a core goal of many Ayurvedic treatments, as it is seen as the root of many diseases.

***ayu.*** Life or lifespan, including body, senses, mind, and soul. Ayurveda aims to prolong lifespan and enhance quality of life by promoting health and balance in all areas of life.

**Ayurveda.** The traditional Indian system of medicine that has evolved over thousands of years. The term comes from the Sanskrit words *ayu* (life) and *veda* (knowledge), meaning "the knowledge of life." Its goal is to promote harmony between body, mind, and soul and to prevent disease.

***dhatus.*** The seven bodily tissues: *rasa* (plasma), *rakta* (blood), *mamsa* (muscle), *meda* (fat), *asthi* (bone), *majja* (marrow), and *shukra* (reproductive tissue). These form the structural and functional units of the body and must be well nourished to maintain health.

***dinacharya.*** The daily routine recommended in Ayurveda to promote health and well-being. It includes practices like waking up early, tongue scraping, oil pulling, and having regular meals. A consistent routine helps maintain doshic balance.

***doshas.*** The three fundamental bioenergetic forces in the body: Vata, Pitta, and Kapha. They govern all physiological and psychological functions. Balance among the doshas is key to health; imbalance can lead to disease.

**Kapha.** Composed of the elements water and earth, it provides stability, structure, and lubrication to the body. It governs immunity and physical strength. An excess of Kapha can lead to weight gain, lethargy, and lymphatic congestion.

***manas.*** The mind, which plays a central role in Ayurveda. It governs perception, thought, and emotion. A balanced mind is essential for overall health. Mental well-being is supported through practices like meditation and mindfulness.

***marma.*** Vital energy points used in massage and therapeutic treatments to support healing and energy flow. There are 108 major marma points, considered intersections of body and mind, and they are key to restoring balance.

***nadis.*** Subtle energy channels through which prana (life force) flows. There are thousands of nadis in the body; the three main ones are Ida, Pingala, and Sushumna, which run along the spine and regulate energy flow.

***ojas.*** The subtle essence of all the dhatus and the source of vitality, immunity, and resilience. It supports mental clarity and emotional stability. A lack of ojas can result in fatigue and vulnerability to disease.

***panchakarma.*** A comprehensive Ayurvedic detox and rejuvenation program consisting of five main therapies: *vamana* (therapeutic emesis), *virechana* (purgation), *basti* (medicated enemas), *nasya* (nasal cleansing), and *raktamokshana* (bloodletting). It aims to remove deep-seated toxins, restore doshic balance, and promote vitality, and is usually personalized and supervised by an Ayurvedic physician.

**Pitta.** Made up of the elements fire and a little water, it governs metabolism, digestion, and body temperature. It is responsible for transformation and energy production. Pitta imbalance can cause inflammation, acid reflux, and irritability.

***prakriti.*** A person's natural constitution, determined at birth. It represents the inherent doshic balance and influences physical and mental traits. Understanding one's prakriti is key to creating individualized health strategies.

**prana.** The life force energy that flows through the breath and the body's subtle energy channels (nadis). It animates all physical and mental functions. Free-flowing prana is essential for health and vitality; blockages can lead to disease.

***rajas.*** A quality of activity, restlessness, and passion in the mind. When excessive, it leads to ambition, desire, and dissatisfaction. It is increased by a hectic lifestyle and stimulating foods and should be balanced.

***rajasic.*** Qualities or foods that promote activity and restlessness. Rajasic foods like coffee, spicy foods, and sugar can increase stress and agitation and should be consumed in moderation.

***rasa.*** "Taste," a key concept in Ayurvedic nutrition. There are six tastes: sweet, sour, salty, bitter, pungent, and astringent. Each affects the doshas differently, and a balanced diet includes all six.

***rasayana.*** Rejuvenation therapies and herbs that promote longevity, youthfulness, and vitality. They strengthen immunity, enhance clarity, and support cellular regeneration. Rasayana is often used after panchakarma for maximum benefit.

***ratricharya.*** Ayurvedic evening and nighttime routines that support restful sleep and overall health. It includes having light evening meals, avoiding heavy or stimulating foods, and doing calming activities like meditation or reading. Its goal is to calm the mind and prepare the body for deep rest.

***ritucharya.*** Seasonal routines that guide adjustments in diet and lifestyle based on seasonal changes. Each season requires specific practices to maintain doshic balance and prevent seasonal illness.

***sattva.*** A state of purity, clarity, and harmony in the mind. It fosters wisdom, love, and peace, and it supports mental and spiritual development. Sattva is cultivated through balanced diet, meditation, and a conscious lifestyle.

***sattvic.*** Qualities or foods that promote clarity, purity, and harmony. Sattvic foods like fresh fruits, vegetables, nuts, and seeds support both physical and mental health and are central to Ayurvedic nutrition.

***srotamsi.*** The channels or pathways in the body through which nutrients, fluids, and waste move. A smooth flow in the srotas is essential for health; blockages can lead to disease.

**tamas.** A state of inertia, darkness, and ignorance in the mind. When dominant, it leads to laziness, depression, and destructive tendencies. It is increased by poor diet, excess sleep, and negative emotions.

***tamasic.*** Qualities or foods that promote heaviness, ignorance, and stagnation. Tamasic foods like processed food, alcohol, and greasy meals contribute to lethargy and should be minimized.

***tejas.*** The inner radiance or brilliance that arises from healthy agni. It supports intelligence, vitality, and mental clarity. Tejas is important for spiritual and psychological growth and is nourished through balanced living.

**Vata.** Composed of the elements air and ether, it governs all movement in the body—including breath, circulation, the nervous system, and nutrient transport. Imbalanced Vata can lead to anxiety, dryness, and constipation.

***vikriti.*** The current state of the doshas, influenced by diet, lifestyle, environment, and emotions. It represents an imbalance from the original prakriti and helps indicate health issues. Ayurvedic treatment aims to return vikriti to prakriti.

# Notes

## 1. What Is Ayurveda Today?

1. Traditionally Ayurveda developed into eight branches (Ashtanga Ayurveda). This classification exists even today:
    1. *Kayachikitsa* (internal medicine) deals with the diagnosis and treatment of diseases affecting the body and mind.
    2. *Shalya Tantra* (surgery) deals with surgical procedures to treat various diseases.
    3. *Shalakya Tantra* (ear, nose, and throat; and ophthalmology) deals with the diagnosis and treatment of diseases related to the eyes, ears, nose, and throat.
    4. *Kaumarabhritya* (pediatrics) deals with the health care of children, including physical, mental, and emotional development.
    5. *Bhuta Vidya* (psychiatry) deals with the diagnosis and treatment of mental disorders.
    6. *Agada Tantra* (toxicology) deals with the diagnosis and treatment of toxic effects of poisons and other harmful substances.
    7. *Vajikarana* (virology) deals with the diagnosis and treatment of sexual disorders and infertility.
    8. *Rasayana* (rejuvenation and geriatrics) emphasizes the promotion of longevity, vitality, and rejuvenation, and encompasses practices that slow down the aging process.

## 2. The Matrix of the Universe

1. Robert E. Svoboda, *Ayurveda: Life, Health and Longevity* (Ayurvedic Press, 2015).
2. *Charaka Samhita, Sustrasthana*, 20.9–11.

## 4. HACK 1: FLOW

1. Wamidh H. Talib, Ahmad Riyad Alsayed, Alaa Abuawad, Safa Daoud, and Asma Ismail Mahmod, "Melatonin in Cancer Treatment: Current Knowledge and Future Opportunities, *Molecules* 26, no. 9 (April 25, 2021): 2506, doi:10.3390/molecules26092506.
2. Annette van Maanen, Anne Marie Meijer, Kristiaan van der Heijden, and Frans

J. Oort, "The Effects of Light Therapy on Sleep Problems: A Systematic Review and Meta-Analysis," *Sleep Medicine Reviews* 29 (October 2016): 52–62, doi:10.1016/j.smrv.2015.08.009.

3. Dental research has shown that approximately 85 percent of all cases of halitosis (chronically bad breath) have their origin in the mouth, which is caused by bacterial residues in the tongue coating. Tongue scraping significantly reduces oral bacteria in the crevices of the tongue and was found to be important for halitosis management. Trent L. Outhouse, Zbys Fedorowicz, James V. Keenan, and Rashad Al-Alawi, "A Cochrane Systematic Review Finds Tongue Scrapers Have Short-Term Efficacy in Controlling Halitosis," *General Dentistry* 54, no. 5 (September 2006): 352–684.
4. P. Stirpe, M. Hoffman, D. Badiali, and C. Colosimo, "Constipation: An Emerging Risk Factor for Parkinson's Disease?" *European Journal of Neurology* 23, no. 11 (November 2016): 1606–13, doi:10.1111/ene.13082.
5. The Colorado-based Ayurvedic physician John Douillard, who used to coach the New Jersey Nets NBA team, elaborates on this in his fantastic book, *Body, Mind, and Sport: The Mind-Body Guide to Lifelong Health, Fitness, and Your Personal Best* (Harmony Books, 2018).
6. Wim Hof, also known as "the Iceman," is a Dutch extreme athlete who developed and popularized a method of breathing and cold exposure that has been researched and shown to improve physical and mental health and stress resilience. The Wim Hof method is simple and widely accessible. It involves a combination of breathing exercises, exposure to cold temperatures, and meditation. Hof is known for his ability to withstand extreme cold and has set several world records for endurance in cold environments, especially ice baths. He has also climbed Mount Everest in shorts and has run a marathon in the Arctic Circle.
7. For more information on intermittent fasting (IF) from a yogic and Ayurvedic perspective, check out the episode "Fasting for Purpose, Clarity and Ambition" from *Thrive with Cate Stillman Podcast* at https://catestillman.com/fasting-for-purpose-clarity-and-ambition-with-cate/.
8. For those interested, please check out the neuroscientist and sleep expert Matthew Walker's fantastic book, *Why We Sleep: Unlocking the Power of Sleep and Dreams* (Scribner, 2017), which sheds new light on why we should pay a lot more attention to the duration and quality of our sleep.
9. We can correlate this with the accumulation of the neuromodulator adenosine, which slowly accumulates in the brain the longer we stay awake, causing us to feel more and more tired. During sleep, adenosine is efficiently cleared from the brain, which is why we feel more refreshed and alert after a good night's sleep.
10. The glymphatic system is thought to be particularly important for clearing beta-amyloid, a protein that accumulates in the brains of people with Alzheimer's disease. Some studies have shown that disrupted sleep may impair glymphatic system function and contribute to the development of dementia and Alzheimer's disease.
11. Dream yoga is a fascinating practice that originates from the Tibetan Buddhist

tradition and involves the use of lucid dreaming as a tool for spiritual practice and self-transformation. In this practice, practitioners train themselves to become aware and conscious within their dreams so they can explore the nature of mind and reality more deeply.

12. Leena Tähkämö, Timo Partonen, and Anu-Katriina Pesonen, "Systematic Review of Light Exposure Impact on Human Circadian Rhythm," *Chronobiology International* 36, no. 2 (February 2019): 151–70, doi:10.1080/07420528.2018.1527773.
13. Erica Sharpe et al., "A Closer Look at Yoga Nidra- Early Randomized Sleep Lab Investigations," *Journal of Psychosomatic Research* 166 (March 2023): 111169, doi:10.1016/j.jpsychores.2023.111169.

## 5. Hack 2: Transform

1. In the *Rigveda*, one of the oldest Vedic texts, Agni is mentioned more than two hundred times, making him one of the most prominent deities in the text. Agni is also frequently mentioned in the other three Vedas: the *Yajurveda*, the *Samaveda*, and the *Atharvaveda*.
2. Alessio Fasano, "Zonulin and Its Regulation of Intestinal Barrier Function: The Biological Door to Inflammation, Autoimmunity, and Cancer," *Physiological Reviews* 91, no. 1 (January 2011): 151–75, doi:10.1152/physrev.00003.2008; Anna Christovich and Xin M. Luo, "Gut Microbiota, Leaky Gut, and Autoimmune Diseases," *Frontiers in Immunology*, June 27, 2022, doi:10.3389/fimmu.2022.946248.
3. In India and other parts of Asia where people eat with their hands, this process starts even earlier, when your fingers touch the food and feel its texture, temperature, and shape. This information is communicated to your brain before you even put a single bite in your mouth.
4. Sara Santa-Cruz Calvo and Josephine M. Egan, "The Endocrinology of Taste Receptors," *National Review of Endocrinology* 11, no. 4 (April 2015): 213–27.
5. Robert Svoboda, *Prakriti: Your Ayurvedic Constitution* (Sadhana Publications, 1998), 62.
6. Masihollah Shakeri et al., "Toxicity of Saffron Extracts on Cancer and Normal Cells: A Review Article," *Asian Pacific Journal Cancer Prevention* 21, no. 7 (July 2020): 1867–75, doi:10.31557/APJCP.2020.21.7.1867.
7. Leila Hamzehzadeh et al., "The Versatile Role of Curcumin in Cancer Prevention and Treatment: A Focus on PI3K/AKT Pathway," *Journal of Cellular Physiology* 233, no. 10 (October 2018): 6530–37, doi:10.1002/jcp.26620.

## 6. Hack 3: Regenerate

1. The seven dhatus are:
    1. *Rasa* (Plasma): Rasa is the first dhatu, which is formed after digestion of food and considered the most important, responsible for nourishing all other dhatus. Its key function is described as *prenanam*, "nourishing."

2. *Rakta* (Blood): Rakta is responsible for providing nutrition and oxygen to all organs and cells. Its key function is described as *jivanam*, "vitalizing."
3. *Mamsa* (Muscle): Mamsa is responsible for providing strength and support to the body. Its key function is described as *lepanam*, "plastering."
4. *Meda* (Fat): Meda is responsible for lubricating the body, providing energy, and protecting the organs. Its key function is described as *snehanam*, "lubricating."
5. *Asthi* (Bone): Asthi is responsible for providing support, structure, and protection to the body. Its key function is described as *dharanam*, "supporting."
6. *Majja* (Marrow): Majja is responsible for producing blood and providing support to the nervous system. Its key function is described as *pooranam*, "filling out."
7. *Shukra* (Reproduction): Shukra is responsible for reproduction and sexual health. Its key function is described as *prajananam*, "reproducing."

According to Ayurveda, maintaining balance and health of the dhatus is crucial for overall resilience and well-being. Any imbalance in the dhatus (along with ama and aggravated doshas) paves the way to disease.

2. The nine prime emotions according to Vedic philosophy are:
    1. Love (*sringara*)
    2. Joy (*hasya*)
    3. Wonder (*adhuta*)
    4. Courage (*vira*)
    5. Peace (*shanta*)
    6. Compassion (*karuna*)
    7. Anger (*raudra*)
    8. Fear (*bhayanaka*)
    9. Disgust (*vibhasta*)
3. Interestingly, *rasavaha srotas* (the channel related to rasa that travels throughout the body carrying lymph) has its root and origin in the heart.
4. Habib Yaribeygi et al., "The Impact of Stress on Body Function: A Review," *EXCLI Journal* 16 (July 21, 2017): 1057–72, doi:10.17179/excli2017-480.
5. Luigi Ferrucci and Elisa Fabbri, "Inflammageing: Chronic Inflammation in Ageing, Cardiovascular Disease, and Frailty," *Nature Reviews Cardiology* 15, no. 9 (September 2018): 505–22, doi:10.1038/s41569-018-0064-2.
6. The concept of the heart-mind is rooted in various spiritual and Eastern philosophical traditions. It refers to the idea that the heart possesses its own intelligence or wisdom beyond the cognitive functions of the brain. In this context, the heart-mind is considered a source of intuitive knowing, emotional intelligence, and spiritual awareness.
7. Eunsoo Won and Yong-Ku Kim, "Neuroinflammation-Associated Alterations of the Brain as Potential Neural Biomarkers in Anxiety Disorders," *International Journal of Molecular Sciences* 21, no. 18 (September 2020): 6546, doi:10.3390/ijms21186546.
8. The churning of the ocean of milk, also known as *samudra manthan*, is a well-known myth in Hinduism, and it is narrated in several ancient Hindu texts,

including the Puranas and the *Mahabharata*. The story goes that the gods and the demons were once fighting over a pot of nectar that granted immortality. To settle the dispute, they decided to churn the ocean of milk to produce the nectar. As the churning began, many divine and mythical objects emerged from the ocean, including the goddess of wealth, Lakshmi, and the celestial physician, Dhanvantari, who brought with him the pot of nectar. Ultimately the gods were able to secure the pot of nectar and defeat the demons.

The churning of the ocean of milk is a significant myth in Hinduism, and it is often seen as a metaphor for the challenges and obstacles that one must overcome on the path to enlightenment.

9. Alex B. Speers, Kadine A. Cabey, Amala Soumyanath, and Kirsten M. Wright, "Effects of *Withania somnifera* (Ashwagandha) on Stress and the Stress-Related Neuropsychiatric Disorders Anxiety, Depression, and Insomnia," *Current Neuropharmacology* 19, no. 9 (2021): 1468–95, doi:10.2174/1570159X19666210712151556.
10. Neetu Singh et al., "Review on Anticancerous Therapeutic Potential of Withania somnifera (L.) Dunal," *Journal of Ethnopharmacology* 270 (April 24, 2021): 113704, doi:10.1016/j.jep.2020.113704.
11. Shankar Mondal, Bijay R. Mirdha, and Sushil C. Mahapatra, "The Science Behind Sacredness of Tulsi (*Ocimum sanctum Linn.*)," *Indian Journal of Physiology and Pharmacology* 53, no. 4 (October–December 2009): 291–306, https://pubmed.ncbi.nlm.nih.gov/20509321/.
12. Usharani Pingali and Chandrasekhar Nutalapati, "Shilajit Extract Reduces Oxidative Stress, Inflammation, and Bone Loss to Dose-Dependently Preserve Bone Mineral Density in Postmenopausal Women with Osteopenia: A Randomized, Double-Blind, Placebo-Controlled Trial," *Phytomedicine* 105 (October 2022): 154334, doi:10.1016/j.phymed.2022.154334.
13. Carlos Carrasco-Gallardo et al., "Can Nutraceuticals Prevent Alzheimer's Disease? Potential Therapeutic Role of a Formulation Containing Shilajit and Complex B Vitamins," *Archives of Medical Research* 43, no. 8 (November 2012): 699–704, doi:10.1016/j.arcmed.2012.10.010.

## 8. The Ayurveda 2.0 Journey

1. Cortisol levels are typically high in the morning, peaking within the first hour or two after waking. By waiting to consume coffee, you allow your body's cortisol levels to naturally decrease, which can support a more balanced energy level throughout the day.
2. Michael Pollan is a famous American journalist and author, best known for his insightful writings on food, nutrition, and the food and agriculture industry. Among his books are *The Omnivore's Dilemma: A Natural History of Four Meals* (Penguin Press, 2007), *In Defense of Food: An Eater's Manifesto* (Penguin Press, 2009), and most recently, *This Is Your Mind on Plants* (Penguin Press, 2022).

# Index